HOW I MANAGE DIABETES

with CGM Power

My Diabetic Journey and How Continuous Glucose Monitors Changed Everything

Lorena Angell

Disclaimer Notice

TABLE OF CONTENTS

FORWARD

by Lisa Zylstra, MS PA-C

Over the past nineteen years I have had the pleasure of working with many wonderful patients in my job as a Physician's Assistant. I offer medical advice from my training and experience but also strive to collaborate with my patients and want to involve them with decision-making regarding their care. When I first met Lorena, I found her to be credible and determined in many areas of her life. I quickly learned how highly motivated she was when it came to her health.

I remember her being frustrated with her blood sugar and I clearly recall the day she requested a prescription for Free-Style Libre, a type of continuous glucose monitor. At the time, I had not been in the habit of routinely prescribing CGM's for my patients with mild or moderately elevated hemoglobin A1cs, assuming it was only necessary in patients with poorly controlled diabetes.

I also recall our discussions when she followed up with me and expressed her excitement and relief that by using the CGM she could easily track her blood sugar levels and see the effect of certain foods. She was so pleased to have real time knowledge of how foods were affecting her, and I was pleased to be able to review the trends and detailed information on the app. I remember discussing with her the passion that she had for this new technology. Her excitement about the product was significant and she wanted to share with me how it could also help my other patients.

I have since been prescribing continuous glucose monitors regularly for my qualifying patients and have had only positive feedback. The ability to easily monitor glucose levels and trends instead of taking the time to frequently use finger stick glucometer checks has been a wonderful tool in the battle against diabetes. I still recommend double checking abnormal readings with standard glucometer testing, but the ease and reliability of these monitors is quite remarkable.

I believe that CGMs can really help patients take responsibility for their choices and see the consequences of their diet. Making healthy lifestyle and diet changes may help avoid potential side effects and costs of medications. On the other hand, sometimes patients are convinced that limiting sweets is all that they need to do to control their diabetes, but these monitors can inform a patient if they really do need medication. And, when medications are necessary, the monitors can evaluate for low glucose readings and the built-in alarms are a helpful safety tool.

I am so pleased to recommend this book and encourage everyone to take an active role in their health and to strive for a better understanding on how our lifestyle and diet choices affect our well-being.

--Lisa Zylstra, MS PA-C

INTRODUCTION

This may seem like a strange way to start a book about diabetes, but without the following incident, I may never have learned about my own health issues.

In February 2007, at forty-four years of age, my husband Larry had a heart attack.

Thankfully, Larry survived, and a stent was successfully inserted into his LAD artery, which opened his blockage. He narrowly avoided open heart surgery. When the doctor came to talk to Larry following the procedure, he said the bloodwork results showed Larry's hemoglobin A1c sat at 5.5%, which put him at risk of becoming insulin resistant or prediabetic. Because of his heart issues, Larry needed to get his A1c under control to prevent future diabetes-related heart conditions.

I remember thinking, *wait, what? Diabetes?* How could Larry have prediabetes? No one in his family had it—not like mine.

At that moment in time, my mother was diabetic, and my grandmother (her mother) had died from diabetes complications. All my life up to that moment with Larry, I had been semi-conscious of the fact that I was most likely predisposed to getting diabetes later in life and was somewhat determined to prevent it. I ate decently and exercised. I kept an eye on carbs and sugars for the most part, and I was only fifteen pounds overweight, according to my doctor.

After Larry's diagnosis, the shock settled in of the deadly bullet he had dodged. We knew we needed to make some drastic changes to our eating habits to help his health. But also, because these changes would be beneficial to both of us and our children who inherited our genes.

Along with the dietary changes, I decided to make a doctor's appointment to get my own A1c checked to establish a baseline moving forward. I was thirty-six years old at the time.

On the day of my appointment, I can remember leaving the house with optimism. I planned to do some grocery shopping after the appointment to buy a long list of foods for Larry's new heart-healthy diet. After feeling like we'd been given a second chance, I planned to approach this new diet plan with full ambition. Plus, as I mentioned, this would benefit me and the kids, too.

I recall sitting in the sterile environment of the exam room, awaiting the results of my fingerstick blood test. *Even though I don't have any symptoms, this is a good thing I'm doing, establishing a baseline,* I kept telling myself. Then the doctor entered the room with my chart.

"Well, you have an A1c of 5.9%. You have insulin resistance. You are prediabetic."

What? My percentage is **higher** *than Larry's?* I felt like someone had punched me in the gut and yanked the rug out from under my feet. This couldn't be right.

The doctor continued talking as my mind spun mercilessly. He said my body wasn't accepting insulin very well anymore and that I needed to take a medication called metformin, which is generic for Glucophage, to help get the glucose out of my blood and into my cells. What's more, I remember how he stated this information with what sounded like a scripted, well-practiced monologue.

The scene is still so vivid in my memory. I remember the doubt that invaded my mind. *No way am I prediabetic, I feel fine.* I didn't have the protruding diabetic belly like my mother or grandmother. I didn't have the classic symptoms of frequent urination or incessant thirst. *The diagnosis has to be wrong, or the testing equipment must be broken,* I thought, trying to rationalize the situation.

When the doctor asked if I had any questions, words tumbled from my mouth with, "How can this be right? I don't eat a lot of sweets. I get over 12,000 steps a day at my job. I feel fine." If I could prove to him that my diet and daily activity excluded me from the diagnosis, he'd reevaluate.

Instead, he flipped a few pages in my chart and stared at them for a minute. "Well, you've marked here that your mother and your maternal grandmother are diabetic. You inherited genes and body type from them, making you pre-disposed."

"Yes, but diabetes is something old people get. I'm only thirty-six."

His reply went something like this: Not necessarily. Type 2 diabetes develops when an abundance of carbohydrates is consumed over a long period of time, causing the pancreas to work overtime and eventually wear out. Insulin production slows and blood glucose levels increase. By the time someone gets old, as you say, and needs insulin, they've had previous years if not decades of elevated A1c levels. Adult-onset diabetes doesn't just happen overnight. But you're catching this early and there's still a lot we can do to get this under control. You need to look at your dietary habits and make changes. Less sugar, less carbohydrates. Then you can slow or even stop the progression of diabetes.

My mind raced. I still couldn't quite process his words as truth. And I didn't want to start some sort of medication if all I had to do was drink a few less sodas.

I told the doctor that my husband and I were changing our diets dramatically because of his heart attack. I asked if I could try to lower my A1c with healthy eating before starting metformin. He agreed, telling me to come back in three months to recheck my A1c, and then handed me the little square paper with barely legible writing. I could make out lowercase letters: i, q, and d.

Following the appointment, I drove directly to the grocery store with the prepared list for Larry's heart healthy diet and a running inventory of what was at home in the refrigerator that I could eat. With my new diagnosis, I needed to consider that this diet wasn't just for him, now. It was for both of us.

I roamed the aisles looking at the foods I would normally put in the cart and with each step feelings of doom consumed me. These were all foods *I* could no longer eat. One box after another, one bag after another, all things I couldn't eat if I was going to reduce my A1c in three months. I felt so disheartened, still confused by my diagnosis.

And a bit angry.

Why was my A1c higher than Larry's? We both drank a lot of sugary soda, but his dietary habits were much worse than mine.

He ate a lot of individually wrapped snack cakes, cookies, and donuts. (Possibly a large contributor to his heart attack.) I didn't have as many sugary treats in my day-to-day diet to eliminate. His changes over the next three months would be much more dramatic than mine, which also meant his results in three months would probably be better because of all the "bad" foods he'd be eliminating from his daily diet. But I didn't eat like he did. So how would I drop my A1c if I wasn't eating a lot of sugar?

* * *

At thirty-six years old, my world crumbled down around me. My fears of becoming diabetic, like my mother and her mother, were becoming a reality, one that I didn't think would happen. My A1c was 5.9%. I was already insulin resistant. Prediabetic. I was only about fifteen pounds overweight, led an active life chasing after daycare children, ate a rather healthy diet—well, except for my caffeinated sugar soda—so how had this come to be?

Not only that, what did my future look like? Would I end up like my grandmother? Would I have terrible complications like my mother?

I wish I knew then what I know now concerning pre-diabetes and diabetes. It would have saved me a lot of time, I would have had less headaches, and less stress.

I am now fifty-two years old (at the time of writing this book.) My journey over the last sixteen years has illuminated the reality of what a large percentage of people are dealing with at present. When the doctor recited his monologue about diabetes, I was right to assume he'd given that same speech over and over again. I was simply the next patient to get the bad news. But to me, it felt extremely personal.

I imagine your diagnosis was just as personal.

I'm hopeful that by writing this book, I can help others who may be struggling similarly to have some added information, some options, and buoyancy in what can feel like a sinking situation.

I invite you to read on about my diabetic journey and what my life was like before I was diagnosed as insulin resistant. In **Part A** of this book, I'll share my personal history prior to and after my diagnosis of insulin resistant, my struggle to manage my A1c level, along with some complications inherent with diabetes. I'll reveal some of my actual lab report numbers, too, so you can see my ups and downs before beginning to use a continuous glucose monitor (CGM) and after implementation.

In **Part B**, I'll run through what I feel are important tools, techniques, and battleplans to manage diabetes in the My Toolbox chapters.

In **Part C**, I'll share my experiences with my FreeStyle Libre CGM sensor device and the trials and errors on my part, so if you choose this path of wearing a CGM, you can avoid these issues and jump right to leveraging the readings to benefit you and your lifestyle.

Disclaimer about me

I am not a doctor. This book is not to be taken as medical advice. The CGM products I mention, like the FreeStyle

Libre from Abbott Laboratories, do not reduce blood sugar on their own but are to be used as a tool in your arsenal of diabetes management. Any data and findings established through the use of a CGM should be shared with your medical provider for assessment and for therapeutic changes to ongoing medications. I am not an employee of Abbott. I gain nothing from Abbott for sharing my results of their product.

Okay, with that out of the way, let's get started!

PART A

CHAPTER 1: GENETICS SUCK!

Childhood

I grew up in a large family of nine children. I am number four. We lived in the countryside, near a small town in Idaho where the closest business was about four miles away—a gas station called Ma & Pa's.

My siblings and I would play tag, baseball, and other outdoor activities with the neighborhood kids, and we'd ride our bikes all over the place, miles at a time, so there was plenty of exercise in my life as a child.

Most of our meals were homecooked, with very few premade ingredients. Mainstay foods in our home were potatoes, pasta, bread, beans, and ground beef. Chicken or roast beef was common for Sunday dinner, with potatoes, of course, and some kind of vegetable. We grew a large garden every year and we would bottle fruit and tomatoes in the fall. We raised chickens for the eggs and the meat and had other farm animals from time to time, too.

With all the yard work, gardening, taking care of animals, and the outdoor playtime activities, I certainly burned off all the additional calories in my diet. And as soda and candy were only for holidays or special occasions, I would have never thought I would need to watch out for diabetes.

I learned from a young age about two words: **diabetes**—the body's inability to process glucose which keeps blood sugar levels high. The other word was **hypoglycemia**—dangerously low blood sugar levels—which my mother suffered from most of my childhood. I think I associated these two conditions with being overweight, especially in the stomach area, because both my mother and her mother had round waists. The idea that I might someday develop diabetes had been on my mind since my youth, but not so much to entirely influence my eating choices. I was a skinny kid, so I felt I was in the clear. All my siblings were thin, too.

I do recall thinking diabetes was something you caught, like the flu. That's false, of course, but I wouldn't get that cleared up in my head until much later in life.

Around nine years of age, I remember watching my fifty-seven-year-old grandmother whip up a batch of her famous homemade whole-wheat bread, slamming the big ball of dough down on the countertop over and over, stretching and pulling, then slamming it down again. She said that helped to activate gluten. Whatever it was, her bread would always rise high and tasted so good with butter and jam. Maybe it just tasted so good because *she* made it and I got to help.

Part of my memories of watching her make bread was the little timer she always had nearby. When the timer chimed, she'd stop what she was doing, clean her hands, and open her diabetic testing kit. She'd prick her finger with a lancet and test her blood on a little machine. Sometimes she would administer a dose of insulin. I remember thinking that I never wanted to have to give myself a shot.

I was almost twelve years old when the youngest of my family was born. My mother was thirty-nine years old. Unbeknownst to my mother and her doctor, she had developed late-term gestational diabetes, therefore my baby sister's vitals crashed shortly after birth, and she was whisked away to the neonatal intensive care unit (NICU) for lifesaving treatment. It took a couple of days for my sister to recover.

Around the same time when the youngest was born, one of my other sisters began to show signs of hypoglycemia as a toddler, which my mother recognized as such and treated accordingly with something sweet.

Other sugar-related memories include my mother lecturing us about sugared soda. Once my brothers started earning their own money, they would bring home twelve-packs of soda and other "junk" food. I remember my mother lecturing them about how much soda they were drinking and saying, "Do you know how much sugar is in one of those cans? Diabetes runs in our family, so you should not be eating that much sugar."

Since I was thin, I didn't pay much attention to her lectures on sugar, thinking I'd deal with it if I ever had to in the future, especially because she would often have something sugary to counteract her low blood sugar episodes. It all felt a bit hypocritical, but I understand now that I didn't understand *anything* then.

I've since learned that during hypoglycemic events, our brains need glucose to function. When the supply is low, our brain can become foggy and dizzy, or we can get nauseous and tired.

Usually, we realize we need to eat something, but so often what we choose to eat is high in sugar, which then sends our blood sugar levels spiraling up, only for it to crash again a few hours later.

My mom went on this vicious cycle all the time. I saw it first-hand. Her hypo moments would make her tired and she'd go lay down, leaving me in charge of my younger siblings. Or she'd snack on something sweet and have the same tiredness shortly after.

And yet, even with my mother's lectures and health issues, an unfortunate habit during my high school years (way back in the late 80's) was to stop at the vending machines on the way into school. I'd buy a cola and a candy bar to start the day. Breakfast of champions. Then after school, I'd go to my job at Dairy Queen where I received a nice employee discount on all the goodies.

Still, since I maintained my weight, I didn't worry about diabetes.

Entering Adulthood

After I graduated from high school, I moved out of my parents' house and married my boyfriend, Larry. My weight of 118 pounds at that time was at the low end of normal, according to my height of five-feet six-inches, and according to the chart I'd received from Health class my senior year.

Into my marriage, I brought along the cooking skills I'd learned while growing up. Our meals were carbohydrate based with potatoes, pasta, and bread, just like at home. Larry brought the love of rice. Fortunately for us, those staples were cheap, helping us stretch our dollars. Unfortunately, we often made too much food. Not wanting it to go to waste, I'd eat more than I was used to eating, and I quickly put on five pounds.

My first child was born in 1991. The pregnancy was a shock to my system. I would get extreme stomach pains if I went too long without food, so I had to eat more often to avoid the aches. By the end of the pregnancy, I had gained thirty pounds. My baby was born full term and healthy.

I shed the extra weight post-birth over the next seven months, at which time I contracted a nasty virus that hospitalized me for a few days, my weight bottomed out at 120 pounds. Of course, losing weight due to sickness is not sustainable. I quickly gained fifteen pounds in the next few months due to our unhealthy, carbohydrate-based eating lifestyle. Back then we referred to our extra padding as evidence of being happy and comfortable.

I started my second pregnancy at age twenty-one, weighing 135 pounds. During a standard prenatal care visit around month six, the doctor was alerted to my higher-than-normal sugar numbers and ordered a six-hour glucose test. The results came seemingly out of nowhere. The doctor said, "You have gestational diabetes." I remember feeling stunned, in disbelief, then angry at myself for letting this happen. I should have made better eating choices. I should have exercised more. I was devastated, but I felt determined to do whatever the doctor ordered to get my health back on track.

I began walking each day and followed a strict diet plan which proved to be effective. I was able to control my blood sugar numbers and never needed to take insulin or other medication. Once I started this intense regimen, I only gained five more pounds in the last three months of my pregnancy. Some people close to me thought that was unhealthy for my baby, but my doctor was pleased with my ability to control my carbohydrate intake, exercise, and control my glucose. Plus, my baby was growing at the appropriate rate. My baby was born full term, with a healthy weight, and didn't need NICU care, like my younger sister had.

I felt proud to have succeeded in fighting off diabetes. At my post-pregnancy checkup weeks later, the doctor said my sugar levels were back to normal. Feeling rather pleased with myself, I relaxed back into my comfortable eating habits.

Diabetes had nothing on me.

Looking back, I realize I didn't have sufficient motivation to continue watching what I ate after my second baby was born. I was twenty-one years old. I had my whole life ahead of me. I mean, how many young adults think about what they want their life and health to look like at retirement age?

Right around the same time as I dealt with gestational diabetes, my mother was officially diagnosed with diabetes. She was in her late-forties and was hospitalized due to the extremely high level of her blood sugar and the fear of imminent coma. I don't know what the glucose number was, but I do know they administered insulin and taught her how to inject it. Once her sugar levels were back under control, she was released with a prescription for insulin.

Not even watching my mother's diagnosis and implementation of insulin was enough to motivate me to change my ways. I was still riding high, feeling like I kicked diabetes's butt or that it only affected me during pregnancy.

Five years later, my grandmother died after developing peritonitis from dialysis due to kidney failure. Twenty years had passed since I'd watched her make bread in our kitchen. Her death was a wake-up call to the reality that diabetes can end your life.

I sometimes wonder if she hadn't had diabetes, would she have lived longer? I've noticed plenty of people live into their eighties and nineties, even to the century mark.

Early that same year, I became pregnant with my third child. Diabetes was fresh on my mind, now, but I had an eating battleplan. This wasn't my first rodeo, as they say. I don't remember what my starting weight was, but I peaked at 170 pounds, and yet I successfully avoided gestational diabetes. My baby was born full term with a healthy weight. Again, diabetes had nothing on me.

While pregnant, I started experiencing premature atrial contractions (PAC) in my heart. I was told it wasn't "heart disease," and is common to develop during pregnancy. I was told not to worry unless it started happening so often it became disruptive to everyday life.

Author note: I still have this condition. The symptoms are that I suddenly feel like I just got the wind knocked out of me. The sensation makes me cough, and then I feel like my heart has skipped a beat. Sometimes I'll have "episodes" where it happens repeatedly over a few minutes, like the hiccups. Premature atrial contractions are common in older adults. I was only twenty-eight years old when this began. I take a low-dose beta blocker every day to minimize this condition.

One year after my third child was born, I struggled to lose the pregnancy pounds, so I went on a low-fat diet, knowing excess weight can make a person more likely to develop diabetes. I needed to bring my weight down to a healthier level.

My fifty-seven-year-old mother's diabetic health issues around that time were extreme high blood pressure and a hemorrhage in one of her eyes. Diabetic retinopathy. Both conditions were addressed quickly, and she didn't lose all her sight in that eye. She did lose her peripheral vision, and her color perception was damaged. I remember a phone call with her where she shared a comical, embarrassing experience about not realizing she'd put on one black sock and one dark blue. She went into a social situation where it was pointed out by a good friend. We shared a laugh together about the awkward event; however, it's clear to me now the reality hadn't truly sunk in that her vision was forever altered because of high glucose levels. That was over twenty years ago.

Moving forward on my diabetic journey, at age thirty, I began operating a licensed home daycare as a way of generating income. The rigors and stress of chasing after several children all day helped me lose some weight, bringing me down to 150 pounds, the tippy top edge of the normal range, according to the CDC's body mass index (BMI) for my height. But that's where I stayed. I plateaued. It didn't matter that I was getting 12,000-15,000 steps a day. My weight was belligerent.

One of the best perks of running a home daycare was being able to participate in the state food reimbursement program. Basically, the program outlined the types of foods and food groups I had to serve the daycare children, like that of school lunch. This was a welcome change to how I prepared meals for my family, too. By feeding the daycare children the approved foods, my own children also received these healthier, nutritious foods. We started eating additional vegetables and fruit, and drinking more milk, to name a few.

Having healthier food options to choose from at my fingertips was a good thing for me and my family. Unfortunately, I also had more sugared caffeinated soda stocked in the refrigerator because, you know, chasing after kids takes energy, and as I didn't drink coffee, I needed my instant energy.

During my years of operating a home daycare, and being inspired by J.K. Rowling's *Harry Potter*, I began writing out the stories circulating in my head. Something about watching other people's children wasn't ringing true with me and I wanted to do something different with my life. Dreams of making it big with a publisher seemed like an easy way to get out of the daycare business, or at least I thought it would. If nothing else, I was able to disengage each evening from the stresses of the day and enter the fictional land I'd created.

At that point in my life, I felt creative, energetic, healthy, and happy. My life was pretty good.

Around that time, I decided to buy some new running shoes because I wanted to get into shape. My weight had increased a little and I didn't want to go higher for fear of what it would mean for my health, (diabetes always in the back of my mind), so I shelled out the big bucks for name brand shoes with great arch support. But my arches didn't like the design and they rebelled. My heel started hurting one morning; not just hurting but feeling like I was stepping onto a hot knife tip. I remember it vividly because we were in a hotel room about to get ready to go to an amusement park. I would be on my feet all day long, walking miles, but I couldn't put any weight on one of my feet. I didn't know how I would to make it through the day.

I survived the day at the amusement park with non-stop ibuprofen treatment and continuous movement.

After a few more days of walking on my painful foot, I could no longer stand the discomfort, so I went to the ER thinking my foot must be broken. Long story short, I had plantar fasciitis, an inflammatory issue with the tendons in my foot. I was sent to a podiatrist, given a prescription for inflammation, and fitted for orthotics. The culprit was my fancy new shoes.

I only wanted to get back into shape.

I've had many examples like this where I start exercising and end up pulling or straining something that lays me up for days. We once bought an elliptical machine and I wound up with severe knee pain, which is ironic. Elliptical machines are designed to be easy on the knees.

The pain I experienced and still experience when starting a new activity outside of my normal range of motion is more than just sore muscles. I liken it to the pain of an injury, not lactic acid buildup. The soreness I experienced once I got into my mid-thirties was different. And, sure, most people start to hurt more as they age, but again, this was different as the pain and soreness wouldn't resolve in a few days or even a week. In fact, whatever part of my body I "injured" would go on to remain injured or become easily reinjured in the future.

Fast forward one year. While running my daycare, I used the bathroom and discovered I had brown urine. I didn't have any pain, or fever, but I knew this was not good. I remember panicking about needing to go to the doctor but not being able to because of the children in my care. I drank lots of water and stared at the clock for several hours, but every time I used the bathroom, I'd see the same color. Finally, I had my husband come home and watch the daycare children so I could go to the doctor. Once there, a CT scan with contrast was ordered to check for kidney stones. I tested positive for a UTI. The doctor also set me up with a urologist appointment because of how often I had been getting UTIs, but I never heard anything about the CT scan results. I just assumed no news was good news.

I had to wait six weeks to get in with the urologist.

At the urologist appointment, he reviewed the CT scan and asked how long it took me to pass the stone. The *what?* He said I had an obvious blockage in one ureter. A kidney stone. I didn't even know I had a stone. I had no pain. And why wasn't I told following the CT scan?

The urologist said, "You should consider yourself lucky that you don't have as many nerve endings as other people do," and then he ordered another CT scan. Everything was all clear. Well, except for finding a moderate sized cyst on my ovary.

No pain with that, either.

It's not too unusual to be unaware of an ovarian cyst. But this was a little too coincidental that I also didn't have pain with kidney stones. Giving birth to my kids certainly hurt, so maybe all my nerve endings were concentrated in that part of my body. Who knows?

I asked the doctor if gallbladder and kidney stones are related even though I'd already been told they weren't when I had my gallbladder removed two years after my youngest was born. The urologist said they are not the same thing, but sometimes people who develop one will go on to develop the other. That was new information. I went home and researched more on my own. I found some correlation with both kinds of stones to that of diabetes—diabetics are more likely to develop one or both kinds of stones. [4]

But I wasn't diabetic, based on my understanding of symptoms, and the fact that no doctor had recommended I have my sugar checked.

The year our world flipped on end

This brings us to the point in time where my husband had his heart attack. Heart disease runs in his family just as diabetes runs in mine. (Sheeze, our kids are royally screwed genetically.)

Larry's heart attack changed his life, and he was very much affected, in more ways than one, but his story deserves its own book.

Because of his heart attack, I learned about A1c or HbA1c and how it's used to monitor the body's ability to manage glucose levels.

A1c is an average of what blood glucose levels have been in the last three or so months in the bloodstream. It is registered as a percentage: 5.6% and below is normal, 5.7%-6.4% is the insulin resistance or pre-diabetic stage, and 6.5% and up is diabetic.

I wasn't too surprised Larry's number was in the upper levels of normal at 5.5%. As I mentioned earlier, his diet consisted of cakes, donuts, hot dogs, and sugared soda. Even though we had healthy food around the house, he'd still eat his favorite things. I guess we were both like that a little bit. My favorite foods were much different than his and included raw vegetables and

Ranch dip. I always opted for more turkey, mashed spuds and stuffing over pie at Thanksgiving. More food instead of dessert.

Yet, I weighed 150-ish pounds, fifteen or so pounds heavier than my doctor thought I should be. Clearly, I wasn't doing great.

Author note: There's a magnet on my refrigerator with a picture straight out of the 1950s of an overweight, middle-aged woman reclining in a lazy-boy chair. She's wearing a typical '50s style dress and clunky shoes, and her hair is done up according to the style then. The words say, "I wish I was as thin as I was when I thought I was fat." Yeah.

When my A1c result came back at 5.9%, I was shocked. I felt shame and anger, all at the same time for letting my body go downhill. I wasn't diabetic, but I was on my way if I didn't make changes pronto!

We stopped drinking sugar soda and started the South Beach diet to help Larry's heart heal and prevent another heart attack, and I can proudly say, we didn't eat a single potato for four months! That's hard to do when you live in southeast Idaho.

I spent a lot of time researching diabetes, oddly, for the first time in my life. I already knew about the kidney aspect of diabetes, and the nerve pain and sometimes amputations, and I guess I knew diabetes could affect the heart, too, and eyes, like with my mother. But auditory, dental, and mental health complications were new to me. I remember feeling that I'd missed an opportunity to prevent a lot of misery in my life by ignoring the predisposition to diabetes inherent in my genes.

Three months after Larry's heart attack and my prediabetes diagnoses, both our numbers had improved. Larry's A1c dropped by a couple tenths of a percent into the perfectly normal range. I lowered my A1c from 5.9% to 5.7%. Still in the high range. I wish I could say I was happy with my results, but I wasn't. I knew I had struggled to maintain a strict diet and realized I would continue to struggle because our children didn't eat the same foods as us. *(That's something to consider when starting a new diet regime. Not everyone in your household will want to eat what you eat.)* We had other—not so diabetic friendly—foods for the kids and I found myself eating little bits of those.

I went ahead and filled the prescription for metformin on my doctor's advice and gave it a try.

My body didn't like it. After a few dosages, I had a reaction where I felt like I was drunk and underwater, or at least what I imagined it might feel like to be drunk, as I had never consumed alcohol before. I couldn't talk straight, and my motor skills were sluggish. I stopped metformin and told my doctor about my experience, to which he agreed that I stop the drug and continue with dietary restrictions.

I decided to focus on increasing my water intake. Hydration is very important, and I was probably not well hydrated. I consumed way too much diet soda throughout the day just for the caffeine, and not as much water as I should. Also, I researched other beverages with good health benefits. I found both good and bad articles concerning health benefits for red wine, coffee, and assorted teas. Pros and cons for these beverages were weighed and measured, and then compared to the nutritional content of soda. My diet soda had only cons, no pros. I decided to switch over to coffee and tea for the natural caffeine, and red wine for the heart-health possible benefits, with an occasional diet soda, and water being my main source of liquid.

At the end of the year of Larry's heart attack, I decided I wanted to try different types of work and closed my day-care. I dabbled in website design, catered local wedding receptions, worked a short stint at a juvenile detention center, and continued to write my books, querying literary agents to see if I could get published.

I saw my doctor regularly, watching my A1c move up and then down as I recommitted to following a better eating plan. But it was difficult for me to stick to healthy eating while being surrounded by fast food and family parties with huge carb-heavy potluck spreads. Having semi-annual doctor appointments really helped me to keep my A1c numbers under 6%. However, I never dropped below 5.7% with dietary restrictions alone.

Larry, on the other hand, reduced his number to a satisfactory level that pleased his cardiologist. I don't remember what the number was, only that I wished my body would respond as well as his did. We were eating the same diet, drinking the same things, but his A1c was lower than mine.

Frustration and notions of unfairness seeped deeper into my life surrounding diabetes. I began to resent it because I couldn't get a handle on my own sugar levels, and the medication made me ill. What else could I do?

Two years later, at age thirty-eight, I perforated a disk in my back by sitting in a chair for four days typing out a book idea.

The book would go on to become an international bestseller in 2011, so there's that. Was it worth the lifelong agony that I still deal with today? Probably not. The sitting alone wasn't the sole source of my back issues. It was the proverbial straw that broke my back. The other elements were improper lifting habits, persistently poor posture, inflammation, and weight gain which added stress to the back. I was misaligned and the ingredients for the perfect storm of insidious back issues began. The painful event brought about doctor visits, imaging, physical therapy, a round of oral steroids, and finally an x-ray guided steroid injection.

The pain subsided and I felt better, but the oral steroids made me gain fifteen pounds.

Unfortunately, during the next six months I developed carpel tunnel syndrome in both of my wrists due to a new job in a bakery. One would think all my typing over the years would have been the culprit for the inflammation in my wrists pressing on my nerves. Not so. I was fitted with wrist braces and over time the painful symptoms resolved.

Clearly, my body was experiencing inflammatory issues.

A couple years later, I had a bad chest cold and was prescribed more oral steroids to reduce swelling in my airways. I gained fifteen more pounds from that round of medication. Methylprednisolone is well-known for weight gain among other side effects. However, the medication did its job and my airways opened.

As time moved forward, annual or bi-annual doctor visits helped keep an eye on my A1c. I'd fluctuate up and down, never going below 5.7% nor going above 6.2%, but note that my top number had increased.

In mid-2011, I listed three manuscripts online as e-books. Two books of one series, and a standalone called, *A Diamond in My Pocket.* The books took off and *Pocket* raced up the charts, both domestic and international. I started getting emails from fans wanting book two or a follow-up book. So, I focused intently and kicked out book two within four months' time in January 2012.

My creativity was on fire. But this meant more time sitting, switching to an even more sedentary lifestyle.

Looking back, I can see I was headed down a slippery slope. For years I teetered on the edge of healthy and not-so-much, but once my inflammatory issues began, I descended faster and faster, slipping and sliding down that slope.

At forty-two years of age, my family and I moved to Washington. My weight had peaked around 190 pounds. If I tried to exercise, something would pull or strain and I'd be laid up for two weeks or more, plus I had developed exercise-induced asthma, so exercising wasn't possible in my mind.

Therefore, the extra weight remained.

But I couldn't stop writing my books. Their sales brought in income. *Good* income.

Back to the chair I went.

That winter, I developed severe back pain which led to another CT scan. They found I had a kidney stone in my kidney, not the ureter, but determined that the back pain was muscular/skeletal, not kidney stone related as stones inside the kidney don't usually hurt. I found a good back doctor and began physical therapy again. The back pain was different than when I had disk issues. Returning to PT was good to also address my ever-present SI joint pain, too.

Lingering in the back of my mind lay the fact that I had a stone camped out in my kidney like a ticking time bomb. At any point, it could decide to drop.

The following spring, and feeling much better, I released the third book in the series. I went on to kick out book four in December. I was exploding with creativity and ambition. Sure, I was overweight, topping 200 pounds, in the obese category according to the CDC, but my A1c was no worse than when I weighed 150 pounds due to my continued healthy diet. I just couldn't lose weight. I tried different diet plans, would drop ten pounds, regain the ten pounds, and so on. Classic Yo-Yo effect.

My book series gained traction. I even had an inquiry from a movie company about media rights. Super exciting! Together with my editor, who would go on to be my agent, we built a proposal which included the series having ten books in total. I would need to write five more books.

My creativity was ablaze. I could do it, mentally. But, because of my incessant back pain, I struggled to sit for extended periods of time. But how could I stop? Other writers would *kill* to be in this position. I couldn't give up now, just because of my weight and pain.

Several months later, my agent pitched the series at a convention and landed a producer! This was a huge, much needed infusion of hope. My husband and I went into the winter and then the spring riding this wave of excitement, at least I did. Larry was burning the candle at both ends, working two jobs to help fund the added editing costs of multiple books, which had increased our expenses dramatically. Especially since my book sales were steadily declining.

Then we learned the producer had a big company on the hook. If they took it and ran, our money struggles would be over.

Right after this upbeat prospect, Larry burned out physically and needed relief. I released book five at the end of that May and started looking for a part time job so Larry could quit his second one. I was hired at my local Walgreens.

But then the miracle happened. The big producers offered a movie option contract for The Unaltered Series, you know, the book *A Diamond in My Pocket* that messed up my back. With the contract came a chunk of money. We could breathe a little easier, but I kept my part-time job to keep editing money coming in.

My new job brought a lot of body aches and back problems. I looked for a new doctor to be my primary care provider who could cover all aspects of my body and was recommended to an internal specialist's office where I began seeing the Physician's Assistant. (I'll refer to her as my PA moving forward.) Bloodwork revealed my A1c had climbed again to 5.9% and I had gained more weight. Because of the weight gain and family history of diabetes, my PA put me back on metformin. I explained what had happened before and my PA suggested I try again, as sometimes the drug could act differently depending on age and diabetes level.

This time, I didn't protest. I had been battling my A1c for eight years. It was time.

This attempt on the medication was successful. Sure, I had some of the common side effects, but nothing like the first time I tried it.

With all the excitement surrounding a movie option deal, I needed to keep writing my ten-book series, but I didn't have as much time as before, and my energy levels were terrible. Turned out, work in retail was hard.

One of the upsides of beginning a regular medication was the increase of doctor visits. One might not think that is an upside. But when you're fighting blood sugar issues, regular blood testing and guidance is important. My PA was awesome! She was and is concerned with all aspects of my health, making sure I get regular screenings, and she's always looking for the complications associated with diabetes.

After being on the medication for a year, my A1c had dropped slightly to 5.8%. My PA said to stay on my diet and come back in one year because all my other bloodwork numbers including cholesterol looked good. I kept working on book six of my series, but with little extra energy outside work, it was slow going. Plus, my part time job had many weeks where I was asked to work full time, leaving even less time to write.

The next year, at age forty-six, my bloodwork showed 6.1% A1c.

I couldn't believe it. How could that number be *higher? What the hell happened to my willpower?* I thought I was doing really well. Blood insulin levels over 18.6 mcU/ml are considered high according to Quest diagnostics. Mine was a whopping 30.8 mcU/ml. And my fasting glucose came in at 122 mg/dl? How? Normal fasting glucose is between 70-99 mg/dl. It was time to raise my metformin dosage and perform bloodwork every three months. Note that ten years had now passed since learning I was insulin resistant.

Author note: blood glucose measurements moving forward will all be mg/dl.

Three months later, at my bloodwork checkup, my cholesterol numbers all looked good. My increased metformin hadn't given me many side effects, but my A1c was even higher than previous numbers and had risen to 6.2%.

This time I had identified the culprits that led to unhealthy eating decisions: mental fatigue and depression. I think I got lazy about self-care, hoping/expecting the higher dosage of medication would take care of my glucose issues for me. I just wanted the medicine to do all the heavy lifting. That, and I felt depressed that I was losing the battle. All my energy was being used up at my job, leaving very little to aim at my books—books with a film option that was expiring soon *without* a movie deal.

Ironically, my fasting glucose was 98, which was in range. So, here's a great example of why A1c testing can reveal more than a single fasting glucose measurement. If my glucose management issues hadn't been discovered yet, and a blood glucose test was the only test run, a medical provider might have said I didn't have a blood sugar problem because my fasting number was 98. That normal score was only a single snapshot of what my sugar level was that morning. Clearly, with a 6.2% A1c, this meant whatever I had been eating spiked my blood sugar too high and too often over the previous three months.

I recommitted to being stricter with my diet plan and set up my appointment for December. It's incredibly challenging to eat right, though, when you're exhausted and limited on food options because of working at a drug store where food choices aren't the best. That, and I failed to plan ahead and take my own lunch.

Additionally, at the September appointment, my PA became concerned about a couple of moles on my body that she wanted a dermatologist to evaluate. She issued a referral.

Later on, at the dermatologist's appointment, the doctor wasn't concerned with the two spots that brought me into his office; instead, he zeroed in on another—a small, solid-black dot on my forearm, seemingly perfectly round. My PA probably overlooked it, thinking it didn't fit the typical "poster" descriptions of cancerous moles. The dermatologist, on the other hand, expressed the need to have it removed that day. He performed a biopsy, and I went on my way.

About four days later, the dermatologist himself called. (Anytime the doctor is the one who calls, you know the conversation isn't going to be good.) He said the pathologist couldn't rule out melanoma, so to be safe, I needed to have a larger margin of skin removed. An appointment was scheduled without delay and a second procedure was performed. The results showed no progression of cancerous cells. Whew!

The mole had enough of the characteristics of melanoma stage zero to be worried about, so my dermatologist treated it as such, which meant I would need to come back every six months for checkups.

Author note: You might be wondering why I'm including this mole removal story in my book about diabetes. While researching for this book, I searched the internet for "melanoma and diabetes." To my amazement, I found an article posted in 2022 on The National Library of Medicine's website called Diabetes and skin cancers: Risk factors, molecular mechanisms and impact on prognosis. [1] I recommend you read this article to further understand the connection between high blood glucose levels and cancer growth. After I finished reading it, I went and re-examined all my spots again to look for any changes.

November brought a break in the clouds. The movie option contract for The Unaltered Series was renewed for three more years, with a big-time distributor interested in the project. This news helped reinvigorate my drive to finish book six.

December, at my appointment, my bloodwork came back at 6.1% A1c with a 115 fasting glucose. A slight improvement from three months previous, which felt like maybe I was headed in a good direction. However, now my cholesterol registered high, outside the normal range. I was forty-six years old, overweight, and rather sedentary with my only exercise happening at my job.

Following that appointment, I researched cholesterol on sites such as CDC.gov, NIH.gov, and watched several videos of doctors detailing what happens in the vascular system due to ongoing elevated blood sugar which causes damage to the vascular system, allowing collections of cholesterol to create blockages after a while—heart attacks, for example.

My numbers at that time were high triglycerides and low HDLs (healthy HDLs have a high number) My PA prescribed me atorvastatin.

The following spring, I released book six of The Unaltered Series. Three long years had passed since book five came out. I had a new editor, newly redesigned book covers, and increased book sales, but I still had to continue working at Walgreens.

At my next appointment, my cholesterol numbers were normal, controlled with atorvastatin. However, my A1c had further increased to 6.3% with a fasting glucose of 120. Six months had blown by since the previous appointment without me knowing my sugars were climbing. I felt genuinely confused. I had taken 1,000mg of metformin, had stuck to my low-carb diet, and was physically active at work. Why was my body so broken? The creeping A1c number seemed to be unmanageable on my low carb diet; obviously I was consuming too many carbohydrates. I asked my PA what she thought about the Keto diet. She had heard good things and gave me the thumbs up.

I started the Keto diet the moment I walked out of the medical office. My next appointment would be in three months. I was determined to have my next A1c test be lower.

As I drove to the grocery store—reminiscent of the day I found out I was prediabetic—a mental inventory flew through my mind of what foods I already had at home and what foods I needed to buy to follow the diet. I bought my first three days' worth of food and headed to work, armed with a goal and with the right food. No temptations would deter me from following this diet. I had to succeed. I didn't want to become diabetic. 6.5% was so close. I just couldn't allow that threshold to be crossed, not without a fight.

Let me just say, the Keto diet is challenging. It takes dedication. There is no half-way Keto, it's all the way or not at all, because you strive to put your body into a state of ketosis where your liver is forced to turn to burning fat for energy. That can only be achieved by dropping your carbohydrate intake levels below a certain point and keeping them there. My level was less than twenty-five carbs a day to stay in ketosis. If you're unfamiliar with just how challenging it is to consume less than twenty-five carbs a day, consider that one piece of bread contains around nineteen carbs.

I bought a glucometer that also tested ketone levels so I could track my progress into ketosis. What I really needed was for someone to smack me upside the head for not buying a glucometer sooner in my diabetic journey. Eleven years had passed since I found out I was insulin resistant. Eleven! I could have at least known what my fasting sugar levels were for all those years. I think I believed that only diabetics needed to poke their fingers and I didn't consider insulin resistance to be diabetic. Maybe my brain processed the "pre" part as "not quite yet" diabetic.

Three months later in October, at my next bloodwork check-up, my PA was floored with my results. I had dropped my A1c down from nearly diabetic at 6.3% to 5.6%. For the first time in my documented medical history, I was in the normal range. My fasting glucose was 106, a little high, but my cholesterol looked great, other than my HDLs which were still a little low, but considering how much fat I ate with my Keto diet, I was amazed all the numbers weren't off the charts. Additionally, I had lost fifteen pounds.

My next bloodwork appointment would be in April following the holidays. I knew holidays could be rough, surrounded by sugary-sweets and wheat-based goodies, but I was determined.

I could do this.

The following April, with my bloodwork visit right around the corner, I noticed a bump on the bottom of my foot, up near the base of my toes, on the pad between my big toe and second. I couldn't tell if it was a developing wart, or maybe a corn. I picked at it and alarmingly a small shard of glass came out. *What the heck?* I had a piece of glass in my foot and couldn't feel it? How? When did this happen?

I searched my brain for when I had knowingly been around broken glass. Then I remembered. September of the previous year, we took a trip to Idaho to visit family. A glass fell and broke on the kitchen floor, and I was barefoot. My sister had me stay in my spot until she swept up the pieces. I waited, then went and put my sandals on. I never felt anything go into my foot. Six months ago! I'd had this thing in my foot for six months? (Of course, there was the possibility I had acquired it more recently without knowing I was around broken glass. The incident at my sister's house was the only time I could recall.)

I planned to discuss the glass incident with my PA at my upcoming appointment. Maybe she could conduct a nerve test or something. Images of my mother's legs and feet flooded into my mind. She'd lost feeling from the knees down. Her hairless legs had a purplish hue to them, and the skin shined. I didn't want that. Even though I knew my mother's legs hadn't turned purple overnight, I was still scared.

My PA shared my alarm. She had a device in the office to test my sensitivity and I passed every time she touched my feet. This was a huge relief. She concluded the glass had entered my skin in a place with no nerve endings. (Another bizarre "no pain" occurrence.) On the plus side, I had shed another ten pounds, my A1c had held steady at 5.6%, and my fasting glucose was 112, a little high. My cholesterol and blood pressure were good, so following the Keto diet plan had worked well for me.

The months came and went while adhering to the Keto diet, and even though my numbers were doing phenomenally well, I could tell I was becoming depressed. Another holiday season was approaching, and my food options were so limited. Plus, I had fallen into a rut of eating the same foods all the time. I remember thinking that if my blood sugar was mostly managed with my diet and metformin, perhaps I could come out of ketosis and follow a low carbohydrate diet.

I just wanted to enjoy eating again, but in moderation, of course.

So, in November, I started eating a few more carbs, and my body freaked out, almost like it had forgotten what to do with glucose. I remember one night after work I felt like my blood sugar might be low, (my glucometer was at home so I couldn't check.) I picked up some fast-food chicken strips and ate them on the way home. I figured the breading alone would help my sugar. I had no idea what my number was but based on the symptoms that developed on the drive home, like tingling tongue and dizziness, I must have been really low. I didn't think to check my sugar when I got home. I just went to bed.

The next day, I still felt yucky but better than the day before. I downed my morning coffee with cream and went to work.

Once I arrived, and still not feeling better, I checked my sugar. I was 65! What? No wonder I felt so bad. My head was woozy, I felt a little nauseated, and my body trembled. I was having a hypoglycemic event. I then realized that my number from the night before must have been dangerously low.

Author note: I should not have been driving in that condition.

I made a mental note to never again ignore the symptoms of hypoglycemia.

My boss knew a lot more about this than I did as her husband was diabetic. She recommended I go buy some orange juice and drink it down. My sugar should start to come up after fifteen minutes. She was right.

This was my first real hypoglycemic moment where I had a number associated with what I felt in my body.

A couple weeks later, right before Thanksgiving dinner, I used the bathroom and found my urine was dark brown. *Really? Now? With everyone gathered for dinner down the hall?* I took a moment to regroup and run a mental inventory. I didn't have any other symptoms, no pain, no fever. The urine didn't appear to have blood streaks, so maybe that was good? I decided to not tell my family that I was probably finally passing the lingering kidney stone. No need to worry everyone. Hopefully, the stone hadn't grown from before, and hopefully it would be painless like before.

The following Monday, I went to the doctor. I was now experiencing pain but only slight discoloration. I tested positive for a urinary tract infection, and possible kidney infection. The doctor put me on a heavy round of antibiotics, ordered an ultrasound of my kidneys, and later a CT scan due to questions with the ultrasound. The results were good, ruling out some more serious issues, but there was something different . . . the word calcification. This wasn't a stone in my kidney that would eventually pass— (all those years I'd been waiting for my kidney stone to drop) —this was a part of my kidney becoming calcified. Possible beginnings of renal disease. However, the calcification was not affecting the function of the kidney, so I'd just go into a holding pattern to watch and wait. I never got confirmation of why my urine turned brown.

Or what happened to the kidney stone found years earlier.

I took the course of antibiotics and my infection healed . . . and then four weeks later, I started having bad diarrhea episodes, like C-dif bad (clostridium difficile.) Every five to seven days my body would empty. After three episodes of this intense dumping, I asked my doctor for a C-dif test. The test came back negative.

At my February appointment, my blood tests came back as 5.7% A1c. *Bummer.* I'd hit the insulin resistance level again. 105 fasting glucose was fairly decent for me. However, after coming off the Keto diet, my cholesterol exploded. Total cholesterol high, triglycerides high, LDLs high. I would need to step up my dietary gameplan if I wasn't going to do the Keto diet. The chronic lower gut emptying was still concerning, and my PA asked that I keep her apprised of any changes or if it didn't go away.

The next month, Covid19 became a global pandemic. Even though the nation went into lockdown, I still had to go to work because being a drugstore employee meant I was an essential worker. (I'm sure you can recall the intense levels of stress the nation and the world went through during that time.) Whatever was happening in my gut wasn't letting up. Every five to seven days, my body would violently empty, and I would get flu-like symptoms. My PA wanted me to have a colonoscopy, but all elective surgeries and procedures were cancelled due to Covid19.

It took me until that summer to even get a phone consultation with the gastroenterologist. My symptoms were concerning to him, and he said I qualified for a procedure. His office would call me and set up an appointment.

I waited and waited, week after week, still no call. Other people around me were also waiting for medical scheduling call backs so I didn't find this lack of communication to be that unusual, given the pandemic craziness.

That fall, I desperately needed a break from work/life. I had sustained an injury on the job and was attending physical therapy three times a week, which required a lot of driving and hurrying to make it back to work. I had been trying to write book seven of my series, but I was so tired after a long day of work and driving to therapy that I struggled with creativity.

I decided to quit my job and finish book seven. I had a little bit of money saved up to help me float along. If I needed to go back to work later, the door was always open.

This was a tough time for me, emotionally. I knew the movie option contract was expiring once again, and I hadn't heard anything from the producers. Movies in general had halted around the world. There was no reason to believe mine would be any different.

It wasn't.

Much of my energy went out the window with the realization that a movie deal wasn't happening. My books were not selling very well, especially after lockdown when people read for like two weeks straight, then switched over to binge-watching every available streaming service. And the fact that I wouldn't be able to hold a book signing release party, because of Covid, I didn't know how I could justify releasing another book, paying the editing fee, while knowing I wouldn't make that money back anytime soon.

But I had fans. I had emails from people wanting book seven. I'd get emails every week, so the pressure to finish was there. I hadn't had a lot of time to write because of my job, but now I'd quit, so I had all the time in the world, well, except for the three times a week I'd travel to Portland for PT. I could finally sit at my computer and let the creative juices flow uninterrupted.

Sadly, my creative energy was not there. My mental processing was gone. Was it all the pandemic craziness? Or had I run out of ideas? I forced myself to write as much as possible, but the story was all over the board. My editor told me later she didn't know how to break it to me that my book wasn't even remotely ready for release.

She didn't have to. I already knew. I canceled my release date, knowing my fans would not like that. But I wasn't going to publish crap, at least not on purpose.

My health numbers weren't doing well, either. My A1c hit 6.0, with a fasting glucose of 115. My cholesterol was horrible, too. You name it, it was bad. And I still had severe diarrhea. I called the gastroenterologist again to see about getting scheduled. They said too much time had passed and that I'd have to have another doctor's consultation.

Ugh, for cryin' out loud.

Feeling like my creativity was gone, knowing my writing skills were subpar, losing the movie option contract, having the realization that I'm just spending money and not earning, I went back to work at Walgreens for the holiday season.

As the first year of the pandemic ended, my back pain had improved enough to be pulled out of physical therapy, and I had an upcoming colonoscopy scheduled in February, along with my next bloodwork appointment.

In February 2021, I had two large polyps (the kind that can become cancerous) removed during my colonoscopy but nothing else was found that could explain my extreme diarrhea. I felt relieved to not have major bowel diseases or disorders, but concerned there was no real explanation for what I had been going through for a whole year.

Following the colonoscopy, my gut settled down and the diarrhea went away. Maybe all I needed was an official medicated clean-out to reset the flora in my pipes. Whatever caused the problem resolved itself, and for that I was grateful.

My bloodwork from that month though...

Agh, cheese-n-crackers! My A1c hit 6.2% with a fasting glucose of 127. My triglycerides, HDL, and LDL levels were all in bad ranges. My PA recommended I increase my metformin again. She had some Xigduo samples (a combination of metformin and Farxiga—a medication that helps you urinate off excess sugars) for me to start.

I do want to point out that I was eating mindfully at that time. I watched my carbohydrates, my sugars, and tried to incorporate fresh vegetables whenever I could, but to no avail. I didn't know what else I could do to help my blood sugar numbers, other than going back on the Keto diet.

At this time, I was given the opportunity to become a pharmacy technician and to learn on the job through the apprenticeship program at Walgreens. It meant better money and a little bit better working schedule that might help with my writing time. I also had the opportunity to learn the "secret" prescription codes the doctors wrote. That metformin prescription from all those years ago with the lowercase i, q, and d meant "take one tablet by mouth every day."

The pandemic was distressing for everyone, pharmacy staff included. Every sniffle, cough, or sneeze was frowned upon and suspected of being the plague. Being prediabetic, I didn't want to catch covid. Diabetes was one of the underlying conditions that caused the virus to be more severe. I got the vaccine as soon as I was able to.

In the pharmacy, I quickly realized learning new things at age fifty was difficult, like how to say ustekinumab or hydrochlorothiazide, and also know what they're used for and the brand names. But I was committed to succeeding at this new job. Oh, but the math. Not my strength. My brain was not cooperating, either. I'd have these moments when what I wanted to say simply wouldn't come out of my mouth. Or something entirely different would come out and my ears would hear it and recognize that wasn't what I was trying to say. The whole experience was surreal.

Not only did I feel like all my writing skills and creativity were gone, but I also had this huge slap in the face that I may not be smart enough to work in a pharmacy. And whatever was going on with my cognitive disruptions had me extremely concerned.

I recall talking to my husband about my feelings, saying I didn't think I could do this. I felt like I was sinking in quicksand, and I couldn't pull myself out.

On top of that, I developed another bladder infection shortly after beginning Xigduo. Turns out introducing sugar into my urinary system causes infections. Who knew? That doesn't happen to everyone. Xigduo works really well in people who can tolerate it. I'm not one of them. I started antibiotics for the UTI and quickly developed a yeast infection, all while not being able to think straight in a high-paced, crazy-making pharmacy setting. Oh, and then my back started to hurt again. My life felt completely out of control, and it seemed everything about my body was broken.

I returned to my osteopathic doctor with weekly visits for back pain where it became obvious that I might be dealing with something more serious. An MRI was ordered of my lumbar spine, the area where I had ruptured my disk back in 2009.

The MRI results showed I had inflammation in and around my L4-L5 (the previously ruptured disk) and other areas of inflammation. They scheduled me for an epidural steroid injection to help reduce the swelling and get the pain under control.

That was it? Inflammation? I felt like I'd been overreacting. No stenosis, no calcification, no nerve impingement. Not that I wanted any of that, I just couldn't believe a little swelling was able to cause so much pain.

One day at work, while venting my frustrations about how hard it is to lower my A1c, the pharmacist asked if I've ever considered using a continuous glucose monitoring system. CGM—like Dexcom or FreeStyle Libre.

My immediate response: "No. I'm not diabetic. I'm not on insulin. I wouldn't qualify."

In truth, I'd interacted with some of the patients picking up their CGMs, asking them what they thought of the devices. The reactions were mixed. But one patient referred to their CGM as a gamechanger for their future. That one stuck in my mind.

Upon further investigation, I discovered a CGM *would* be covered by my insurance. Game on! I decided I'd ask my PA to write me a prescription at my upcoming visit if my numbers had climbed any more.

Diabetes

At my checkup, any ideation I had of controlling my blood sugar was shattered with my bloodwork results. My A1c had jumped to 6.7%, an astounding increase of five tenths in three months, a half of a point, even while being on the increased metformin and Farxiga contained in Xigduo and trying to eat a low carb diet. I had crossed the threshold and was now officially diabetic. Not only that, but my fasting glucose came in at a whopping 140. My blood insulin was out of range also at 22.6.

At age 50, I had officially been diagnosed with diabetes. The feelings of complete loss of control over my body were overwhelming. I had fought this battle for over fourteen years, and I had failed.

I asked for a CGM prescription. I would continue my low carb diet and current levels of metformin and return in three months.

After picking up my FreeStyle Libre14day sensor, and having applied it to my arm (which was a little jarring the first time), I waited for the sixty-minute countdown for the first numbers to come in. I had eaten a small piece of cake within the time frame, so it was no surprise that my sugar level came in at 180. Not good. But I could also see with repeated scans of the sensor that my number was dropping. I became fascinated with my new toy, scanning the sensor continuously, using the corresponding app on my phone. I showed it off to my pharmacist and together we watched my glucose number return to a healthy range over the next hour.

For the remainder of the day, I found having the ability to see my glucose without pricking my finger to be addicting and intriguing. I could even check my numbers through the night. But then it stopped being fun as reality set in. The numbers were real. They showed me how my body responded to different types of foods and drinks.

Earlier that month at my checkup, I was truly shocked by my A1c number. I'd felt like I'd been careful with my diet. I believed I'd been doing good. But now, with the continuous glucose readings, I had to take accountability for my food choices.

I now had a window into my body to show me in real-time why my A1c had changed. I could no longer brush off the occasional small piece of cake as no big deal, or convince myself

I was eating healthily enough. This little device showed me the truth—my body doesn't process carbohydrates well, both simple and complex. I had known it since 2007, but I had never ***known*** it until now. And now I had to own it.

I needed to make changes.

I began experimenting with foods, waiting till my sugar was down, and then eating a measured amount of something. Then I'd wait to see where my number would crest and how far down it would dip until returning to where I began. The process would take at least two hours. That was two hours of not mindlessly eating, because of performing an experiment—and it was revealing. I learned French fries, tater-tots, and hashbrowns were the devil for me. They all spiked my blood sugar horribly. Having eaten potatoes in many forms all my life, I finally saw what they were doing inside my body. I would need to make some drastic changes to my potato consumption habits: such as smaller servings, added protein, and/or greatly reducing how often I ate potato products.

Regarding the issues with my back, the injection took a few weeks to do its job. During that time, I dealt with the side effects of the medications I was taking which included some severe gastrointestinal pain—which landed me in the Emergency Room—and another UTI. Communicating with my PA, she recommended I go off my diabetes medications and let my body calm down while I battled with my infections. She told me to monitor my blood sugar closely and to eat wisely. *No sweat*, I thought. Now that I had my CGM, I felt I would be able to keep my sugars under control while I let my body cleanse.

As a few weeks passed, my infections healed, and my back felt better. Life in the pharmacy was running smoothly, and I felt that maybe I could actually handle the job. However, my blood sugar average began to increase, according to my CGM, even though I was carefully monitoring every bite. I panicked and asked my PA if I should return to taking the metformin. She advised me to do so. I saw the results within a few days. (Note how I was able to monitor my blood sugar and see the rising numbers on an hourly, daily, weekly basis in real time, not three months later when the A1c test numbers came in.)

I began to think that by having the CGM on my arm, metformin in my body, and continuing to make smart food choices I could succeed.

But then a weird thing happened.

Brain Fog

Until it returned, I never knew what I had experienced was termed brain fog. What is it? My brain fog may be different from other people's description. I experienced slow processing, difficulty saying the words I wanted to say, counting pills and forgetting which needed to go into the amber vial and which went back into the original container. Did the sixty tabs go into the vial and the forty tabs into the bottle? Without thinking, I'd do it wrong. Not a life-threatening mistake by any means, but an unhappy customer if they were shorted pills. On several occasions I would catch myself slipping up and would correct the error. But how many times did I not catch the error? I still don't know.

Brain fog also makes it hard to recall information in a snappy manner. For example, I'd speak with a familiar person and just couldn't recall her name. Sometimes I would openly admit I couldn't remember her name due to a brain fart. We'd laugh and she'd tell me. But ten seconds after she walked away, I had forgotten it again.

Then there was my inability to focus on my writing. Book seven was this unattainable conquest, an unreachable summit I simply couldn't get my mind to climb—or even dwell on—or remember where I left off last time I worked on the manuscript.

What was wrong with me? My grandfather had Alzheimer's. Was I developing Alzheimer's?

I've never had a perfect memory, even in my younger years, but this level of forgetfulness was above what was normal for me. I had to stop and think through what was happening in my brain and body. Some combination of diet/meds was causing my brain fog, and my money was on the metformin, even though the list of common side effects didn't mention it.

Using my CGM and a carefully plotted diet plan, I stopped taking my metformin again.

A few weeks went by, and I started feeling more alive. I had an improved ability to focus, and became quicker with my verbal acuity, which is very important in a pharmacy. I also started having more energy and excitement for writing in my books. Fresh ideas began flitting through my head and my vivid dreams returned. Only when they came back did I realize they had been gone for so long. My overall sense of self was returning. My learning progress in the pharmacy jumped by leaps and bounds, yes, even the math.

In late August 2021, my husband and I went on a trip to Idaho to visit family. I showed off my CGM and what it could do. I wanted my mother to give one a try, but she kind of blew me off. My numbers were not good, she pointed out. Even with low carb foods, I couldn't get below 125. I think she misunderstood the concept of the continuous glucose monitor. Perhaps she saw it as a regulator, a medicinal device like an insulin pump, not as a sensor that displays the current blood sugar in real time.

While in Idaho, eating smart was problematic. We attended two potluck-style dinners, one for his family, and one for mine. At Larry's family dinner, there were many choices of favorite dishes contributed by relatives. My contribution was a low-carb dish I'd made several times: Zoodle salad. Zucchini noodles (raw zucchini put through a machine that shreds it into long strands, like spaghetti), with Italian dressing, tomatoes, olives, green onions, bell peppers, and fresh mozzarella chunks. Positively healthy and carb friendly. I remember placing my salad on the table with everything else, sliding the bowl between the potato salad, Jello salad, pasta salad, assorted chips, corn casserole, baked beans, hamburgers (white bread buns), cookies, cake, and soda to drink. I was disheartened as I stared down at all the food provided. With my low carb diet, the only thing I should have eaten was my Zoodle salad and a hamburger patty wrapped in lettuce. But, not wanting to insult my family, I dished tiny amounts of each salad and casserole, and a sliver of cake. I chose water to drink, and ate my beef patty with a fork, no bun.

My blood sugar spiked. I knew it would, due to all the past experiments I had done with my CGM, but I felt I would offend others if I didn't try their foods, especially because they talked them up with excitement, just like I did with my Zoodle salad.

My family's potluck dinner was the same. Carbs, carbs, and more carbs, along with bar-b-qued chicken and my salad.

Following the trip to Idaho, I was happy to get back home, so I could get my sugars under control—well, as much as possible without the help of medication. I'd been wanting to call my older brother, who is a doctor, to share my findings with the CGM, but I hadn't had the time, or when I did, he wasn't available to talk. However, after returning from our trip, I was able to reach him.

I remember the phone call, feeling so happy with the return of my mental progress and sharing the functionality of the FreeStyle Libre with him. I figured he'd appreciate the information in the event he wanted to prescribe a CGM to any of his patients.

On the call, he listened to me respectfully and then dutifully chastised me for going off my metformin. "You have diabetes, Lorena," he said. "Your pancreas is over-worked and if you don't take this seriously, you're on track to need insulin." He said other things, too, like that I needed to comprehend that my cells do not accept glucose as they should, and unless I planned on eating the Keto diet the rest of my life, I needed metformin or something else to help my body, side effects be damned. I had to accept that I am diabetic.

Blankety blank, blank, blank! Ugh! Fine. He was right. I'd go back on metformin.

Like a freight train

Like a freight train barreling down a hill, out of control, my brain fog returned a few days after restarting metformin. My newly emerged creativity died, ripped away like a needle scratching across a vinyl record, and now I knew without a doubt that metformin had been the cause of my slowed writing progress, my lack of creativity, my feeling like I was in mental decline.

I had fully accepted what my brother pointed out: I was diabetic. I needed medication to help my body process glucose, but metformin plus my body equaled unfavorable side effects. There were other options, however, I knew this because of my time working in the pharmacy. I called my brother again and asked for his opinion after explaining what was happening in my mind and body. He gave me a few medication suggestions to talk over with my PA.

My next appointment was a few weeks away. In the meantime, I dedicated myself to eating low, low carb and I stopped taking my metformin again. (I didn't tell my brother.) With my CGM as my constant reminder of how well or not well that was working, I persisted.

Author note: I need to take a moment and give my brother credit for helping me find my proper motivation to manage my diabetes, my "why." His blunt scolding didn't feel good, but it forced me to think about my life and the direction I was headed. Instead of thinking "I don't want to become diabetic like my mom," or believing I could somehow still manage my sugar levels, I brought everything down to a personal level, to my level, *my present, my future, and my choices. What does being diabetic mean for me and my life? What do I want out of the rest of my life? This change in attitude toward the malfunction in my body ironically felt more positive than wallowing around in the "why is my body so broken? It's not fair," mud. By changing my mindset to "what do I want out of life?", I've changed my whole approach to my dietary landscape. So, thanks, bro!*

At the next appointment, my A1c was 6.8%. What a let-down! My A1c had actually climbed another tenth of a point, even though I had been basically eating the Keto diet or low carbs for three months. Yes, I had the off/on/off relationship with my metformin during those three months, so that was part of the problem. Even worse, my fasting glucose was 142. Blood insulin levels were 21 (18.6 and under is normal.) Cholesterol was decent, though. Why couldn't diabetes be as easy to manage with medication as cholesterol?

After explaining my metformin dilemma, and with the knowledge that the SGLT2 inhibitor class of medications hadn't worked for me either (Farxiga), I asked my PA about other possible medications like what my brother had mentioned. Together, we decided to try GLP-1 medications, Ozempic in particular. Now, this was before the hype and craze began around Ozempic. This medication was another one to try in the arsenal of diabetes medications to control blood sugar. Victoza was another possibility, but that one required a daily injection, and I didn't want that, so I chose Ozempic. My PA wrote the prescription, and I began my Ozempic journey with my CGM to guide me.

Ozempic is a once-a-week injection that reduces appetite by slowing the emptying of the stomach, helping insulin levels and glucagon levels operate at better numbers. And of course, it can bring about weight loss. Ozempic is one of those medications that takes a while to build up in the body and takes a while to wane once stopped. A weekly dose creates an optimal consistent level of medication once buildup is achieved. For optimal results, I take it on the same day each week.

There is a whole list of side effects that can happen with this drug. For me, I was already eating small portion sizes, so I hoped I wouldn't have the overfull feeling or the vomiting that others suffered from. However, I had decided going in that I would give this medication my all, unless it caused brain fog.

My body handled Ozempic just fine at first. Maybe a little nausea here and there for the first three weeks, but no brain fog. I was using the FreeStyle Libre2 at that time to track my sugar levels.

After about three weeks of using Ozempic, I started losing weight and having lower glucose numbers. At first, I was like, *Yeah!* Finally, I was under 100 at any point in the day. But then I was like, *Whoa, hold on. Why is my glucose dropping so much? Is this normal?*

At week four, I was supposed to up my dose to 0.50mg as recommended. It's part of titration, slowly building up the drug to the desired level with the least amount of side effects while effectively managing blood glucose levels. My 0.25mg level was sending my glucose down to hypo-glycemic levels and I wasn't sure if I should up my dose, so I called my medical provider. The nurse got back with me and said I should either just stay at the 0.25mg dose or stop taking it all together because it shouldn't be causing hypoglycemia. I chose to stay at 0.25mg for another four weeks and use my CGM to guide me through the lows. The hypo moments lessened, so I then upped to 0.50mg.

I had more nausea at this level than the lower level, but I could tell with the CGM my nausea was not related to hypoglycemia, so I didn't worry about it as much. I stayed at the 0.50mg level until my next appointment.

Because my sugar tended to run low (for the first time in my diabetic life), I found I had to force myself to eat carbs to keep my sugar levels up—a huge change from the Keto mindset. Using the CGM, I was able to see in real time what my blood sugar numbers looked like, therefore I could eat carbs as my sugar dropped to fend off a hypo moment. I had to use careful consideration of what foods I chose to eat. I also took notes in a logbook about which foods were steady sources of energy without the rapid sugar dive.

January brought a fresh new year. Hopefully, a better year. At my check-in with my PA, my bloodwork came back with mind-blowing results. I had dropped a full point from 6.8% to 5.8% in three months' time with Ozempic and using my CGM. I hadn't ever dropped that much with any other method, not even the Keto diet. Plus, I was eating carbs. My fasting blood sugar was 105 (still couldn't get below 100 in the morning), and my cholesterol was good. Blood insulin levels dropped into the normal range as well, down to 16.5.

Additionally, my energy levels were improving, my writing became easier, and I was able to get back to that elusive book seven in my series.

I remember finally feeling whole again.

Fast forward three months, and my A1c had dropped even more, down to 5.5%. I had made it into the normal range. I could hardly believe it. The last time I hit normal was when I was on the Keto diet at 5.6%. But I was also on metformin, experiencing brain fog. Not now, though.

Because my sugar numbers were doing so well, my doctor and I decided to push the next visit out by six months.

In all my excitement about hitting the 5.5% number, which was a huge moment for me, I'd forgotten how Larry's cardiologist had raised the alarm following Larry's heart attack about his A1c level nearing insulin resistance. 5.5% is near the top of the normal range, and it indicates the body's average sugar levels are running at approximately 118, which is elevated. I didn't want to have damage occur in my vascular system because of high sugar levels.

I took Ozempic all of 2022 and managed my diabetes with a careful watch on what I ate. I started to incorporate more carbs in moderation, experimenting with my CGM to see what they did to my sugar levels.

I also found that exercise affected my blood sugar. I once brought on hypoglycemia by climbing two flights of stairs three times in a row, hauling luggage to a hotel room. By the time I reached the top on the last trip, my legs were extremely weak. I could feel the low. Moments later my CGM alarm went off, displaying 53. (Alarms are discussed in chapter 15.) Prior to the stairs, I was 89. I learned that if I'm going to exercise, I need to be prepared for sugar to leave my blood stream. The large muscles, like in the thighs, will use up their stored glucose and then will pull sugar out of the blood to restore strength. I learned I needed to be aware of my sugar number before beginning to exercise. I should have eaten a carbohydrate snack to bring my sugar up a little to offset the drop. I know that now.

In October 2022, even with working full time in the pharmacy, I finally finished and released book seven of my young adult series. Four long years had passed between book six and seven. Because my mind was clear, not foggy, and my blood sugar was controlled, allowing for more energy, I was able to be productive with my spare time and complete the book.

What a relief to have my mind back! Now, if only I could get my lower back to stop aching.

Throughout the latter half of 2022, I began going to a chiropractor along with physical therapy seeking pain relief and to avoid getting another steroid injection. The chiropractor helped loosen my continually stiff neck, and PT worked on my back. Around October, I asked my PA if I could get a prescription for Celebrex, an anti-inflammatory medication, after doing some research about chronic back pain and inflammation. I'm so glad I did. Nearly ninety percent of my pain went away immediately after starting the medication.

December 2022, I switched over to FreeStyle Libre3 which is what I currently use. This model doesn't have a reader. It uses an app on my cell phone to collect data. I only need my cell phone nearby to get the upload—no more scanning my arm, other than when setting up a new sensor. I really like it. However, as of writing this, there isn't a volume control for the alarms. They are either off or on. And they are LOUD. Because of this, I turned off the two programmable alarms.

Consequently, having turned off my upper alarm through December, I found I overate carbs. (Too many easily accessible Christmas goodie plates.) My numbers began to climb due to not being reminded that my food choices were too extreme. I guess I felt more comfortable because my instant accountability reminder wasn't pinging. I really wish the Libre3 had volume control options.

January 2023, after enjoying the holiday season a little too much, I wasn't blindsided to get the results of my A1c: 5.7%. Bummed, to be sure, but not surprised. However, my fasting glucose was 102, which for me is pretty good. That pesky blood insulin level climbed up again to 20.7, but my cholesterol was cruising in the green zone.

Because of not being happy with my backslide, I recommitted to taking much better care of my body. I reevaluated my "why" and my future. It's helped me a lot to do this every now and then.

Concerning my back pain and SI joint inflammation, the Celebrex was working very well. I hadn't needed to go to the chiropractor or PT since the end of November, and the stretches and exercises I learned had so far been able to get me through and keep my pain manageable. Success!

At the January medical visit, my PA said tongue-in-cheek that I should work for FreeStyle Libre or be a rep because my stories and personal examples were stellar and had helped her with other patients. We laughed at the thought, but it did put another idea into my head. I'd write a book about my experience with CGM and my diabetic journey.

And here it is!

* * *

What does the future look like for me? Definitely better than before I started using a CGM. Coupled with my continual healthy eating choices, keeping my appointments with my doctor, and staying consistent with my medications, I feel I'm on a good pathway. If my numbers begin to show that my medications are not as effective as they have been, I'll be able to see it sooner than once every three to six months, so I don't lose too much ground before implementing new therapies.

Diabetes is a condition that I may not be able to reverse, but I can certainly keep it in check through diet choices, exercise, medication, and technological tools such as continuous glucose monitoring systems. I feel I'm in control of my body . . . finally!

Where are you on your diabetic journey? I encourage you to put your timeline together even if it is just dates and test results. When were you first diagnosed? What illnesses or health conditions have you suffered from prior to diagnosis? What are your current and past bloodwork numbers.

I will say, by writing this book and gathering my own data for a timeline, I was able to see my fluctuating A1c numbers on paper rather than in my sometimes-faulty memory. I feel like this has helped to hammer home the need to watch what I eat.

If you are new to glucose management issues, hopefully sharing my story from childhood to diagnosis and on to this point has shed a little light on some of the all-too-common struggles diabetics face.

If you have been dealing with glucose management struggles for a while, I hope my story was relatable and will inspire you to make changes for the future you want to live.

No matter where you are on your journey, know that you are not alone.

The next section of the book discusses what I feel are valuable components of effective diabetes management. My toolbox is something I want to share with you as it has helped me thus far in my blood glucose management. Naturally, continuous glucose monitoring is one of the main components.

PART B

CHAPTER 2: MY DIABETES TOOLBOX

Why do I want to manage my blood glucose levels? According to the CDC's website, diabetes or elevated blood glucose levels can cause complications such as (but not limited to):

- Heart disease
- Chronic kidney disease
- Nerve damage
- Foot health issues, including amputation
- Oral health problems
- Hearing loss
- Vision loss
- Mental health issues

This list has become very real for me in the years since being diagnosed pre-diabetic. Prior to that I kind of dismissed it, thinking these things wouldn't apply to me. Please allow me to break each of these down a little bit. By doing so, I'm hopeful you'll see why the components of my toolbox are necessary for my overall health, and perhaps yours as well.

Heart disease. Keeping on top of my cholesterol and blood pressure is crucial to maintain proper blood flow, which brings sufficient oxygen to my extremities and organs. Those numbers are as important to monitor as my blood glucose levels. Blood pressure checks are part of every appointment with my medical provider, so if a reading is outside the normal range, my PA can address it.

Heart disease can lead to a heart attack or stroke if not treated and managed. I don't want that, and I believe you don't either. If your A1c is greater than 5.7% and your doctor is *not* checking your cholesterol, I suggest you ask them to check it.

Chronic Kidney Disease (CKD) and failure. As with heart disease, cholesterol issues and high blood pressure can result in CKD, which can lead to failure and the need for dialysis. My PA has paid careful attention to my blood pressure, even trying to be proactive by starting me on low doses of blood pressure medication to protect the small veins in the kidneys. With regular blood draws we can determine if the kidney function is still optimal. CKD is a long, drawn-out ailment that can lead to death, as in the case of my grandmother.

Presently, my mother has stage 2 kidney failure due to diabetes complications. I have had several kidney stones and have a small amount of calcification. My hope is to manage my glucose levels and prevent additional damage.

Nerve Damage. Tingling and numbness in the feet is a very common symptom of diabetic nerve damage. Hands and fingers can also have these symptoms.

My mother has no feeling below her knees. I know she has dealt with intense neuropathic pain in the past as the nerves were dying. But at some point in her life, she had feeling and sensation. The transition has been long and slow, which is typical, but no less painful.

In the process of writing this book, I've researched more about diabetic neuropathy and found there are several different kinds of nerve damage, including autonomic damage that can take away your ability to recognize the symptoms of hypoglycemia. The warning signs of low blood sugar are the body's way of preserving itself; the brain sends out these signals to tell you something is wrong. "You need to eat something!" But if the nerves needed for this signal are damaged, no warning is received. Hypoglycemia can be fatal if untreated. (Another great use of a CGM is the hypoglycemia alarm that can alert you or others caring for you that your sugar is low.)

The nerves that control the stomach can also be damaged causing gastroparesis, or stomach paralysis.

Nerve damage can bring about loss of bladder control and losing genitalia sensations.

Another is cranial neuropathy. This nerve damage affects the twelve pairs of nerves that control sight, eye movement, hearing and taste.

The damage high blood sugar causes to the nervous system is pretty scary to me. I've seen it in my immediate circle of family and friends and it's nothing I want. If I can prevent it by managing my sugar levels to the best of my ability, I will.

I encourage you to visit the American Diabetes Association website at Diabetes.org to learn more about the other kinds of nerve damage associated with diabetes.

Foot Health issues. Diabetics need to check their feet regularly. A simple blister can turn into an abscess, which can grow into an unmanageable problem very quickly. Regular inspections are important, especially if nerve damage and numbness are factors. Think about the shard of glass I had in my foot and didn't even know it. I'm still amazed that happened. The nerve issues in my body, or lack thereof, may or may not have anything to do with diabetes. I may never know. What I do know is if I strive to keep my blood sugar under control, I will avoid further blood-sugar-related damage to precious nerves and capillaries in my feet.

Oral Health Problems. Dental checkups are good for everyone but are especially a good idea for diabetics. I'm a bad example of this, but I'm committing to do better as I know high blood sugar affects the white blood cells and their ability to fight infection. Gum disease and root infections are harder to cure in diabetics. I don't want a simple problem to become a major infection or abscess because of waiting too long before an appointment. Just as an infection in a foot can turn extreme, so can a tooth infection.

Hearing Loss. High blood sugar can damage the small vessels and nerves of the inner ear, damaging the connection to the brain. This is different than the cranial neuropathy talked about earlier. Before writing this book, I didn't even know diabetes could affect hearing, so I will be getting my hearing checked soon.

Vision Loss. I try to get my vision checked annually and when I do, I sign up for all the bells and whistles, including dilation. Getting a healthy checkup is rewarding, but so is finding slight changes or evidence of vascular issues before they cause blindness. Even though blindness isn't a fatal complication, I don't want to lose my sight.

Mental Health can be affected in many ways while battling diabetes. Don't brush off feelings of depression due to lifestyle changes. Keep an open channel with your doctor to address anything that surfaces. Speaking from experience, I've dealt with the depression of realizing my body does not work the way I want it to.

I try to be aware of my levels of mental wellness as I face each day with diabetes, and I watch for diabetic distress, which is more about over-worrying about what to eat or what not to eat to maintain healthy glucose levels. (I'll cover more about diabetic distress in the Healthy Eating chapter.)

Other possible complications. Even though skin cancer or any cancer is not listed on the CDCs list, I feel it's important to know elevated blood glucose levels attribute to increased risks of being diagnosed with this malady, as I mentioned earlier. [1]

Financial stress. This complication is all too real. Deductibles and co-pays from doctor visits, tests, medications, and ER visits add up. I see this in real time in the pharmacy when patients struggle with the cost of their medications. Sometimes a patient will only pick up some of their meds and wait till payday to get the rest. I feel horrible knowing there's nothing I can do to help them in that situation.

If you're struggling financially or with insurance coverage, I encourage you to speak with your doctor about which areas would be best for you to focus on. There may be an alternative medication that is less expensive.

By improving the management of my diabetes, discussing my findings, successes, and failures with others who struggle too, or use of medication if needed, I can pull myself forward on my diabetic journey.

I'm optimistic that you are feeling motivated to change your approach to your blood glucose management. I believe a way to help this change be easier and more successful is to arm yourself with a good toolbox of equipment and battle-plans. My toolbox is the term I use to refer to the elements that help me monitor and maintain healthy glucose numbers.

What's in my toolbox, you ask?

- Healthy eating battleplan
- Continuous glucose monitor
- Logbook
- Regular doctor's visits with bloodwork and tests (including dental, vision, hearing)
- Medications
- Glucometer for testing when my CGM is unavailable or inaccurate
- Active lifestyle battleplan and mental health monitoring
- Blood pressure monitor and pulse oximeter

These components will help me prevent or significantly diminish the complications of diabetes, but only if I use them. Simply wearing a CGM won't fix anything, but by seeing the numbers and then acting upon the results, I can formulate a plan of action with my medical provider to address my body's unique reaction to certain foods and medications. This helps keep my blood sugar numbers down and hopefully prevent the development of complications.

Come along with me as I detail out the components and see which sound like they would fit for you.

CHAPTER 3: TOOLBOX ESSENTIAL - HEALTHY EATING

You are what you eat

Healthy eating is the #1 way I manage my blood sugar levels. I hope your doctor gave you dietary recommendations or a specific diet to follow and/or scheduled a meeting with a dietician to help you on your diabetic journey. I will not be recommending any specific diet to you, as I am not a dietician, nor do I know exactly how your body will respond. However, I am a seasoned CGM user and a diabetic so I can share my experiences with you about what I've learned on my journey.

First up, as a pharmacy technician, I've seen plenty of first timers. These are the patients fresh from the doctor's office, having just learned they have high glucose levels. They usually have a bundle of paperwork from the doctor, listing recommended foods, the prescribed medications to pick up, and so on. Sometimes they have already been shopping and I can see the contents of their cart, all healthy food choices. As I ring up their new glucometer, test strips, lancets, and most likely metformin, I wish I could express support, letting them know they are not alone. But as a pharmacy technician, I cannot interact with the patient concerning their medications or health issues as that is the pharmacist's responsibility.

Something positive I've noticed with new diabetic patients is their doctors are increasingly prescribing continuous glucose monitors right out of the gate. This is great! I believe these new patients will have a much better chance of sticking to a new diet if they can see what the foods they eat are doing to their sugar levels in real time. Hopefully they will receive proper training on how to use their CGM to maximize the usage.

Healthy eating for long-running diabetic patients, the seasoned veterans, who want to bring down their A1c, requires evaluating what they're consuming daily. I am an example of this. I had tried to manage my diabetes for fourteen years with diet, medication, and exercise but was losing the battle. If you fall into this category, asking your doctor about getting set up with a CGM may help you identify the foods that are most likely keeping your A1c high. It certainly worked for me.

Whatever diet you adhere to, you'll probably still have cravings for unhealthy foods. I feel there is a balancing act between over-indulgence and extreme dieting. I've done both. What worked for me was finding the middle ground on the seesaw: satisfying cravings without overindulgence while still adhering to glucose friendly foods. The Keto diet was the most extreme diet I've tried, and I adhered to it for over a year and a half with success. But I concluded that I couldn't keep up with that way of eating for the rest of my life, and I stopped. I now have a lot more self-control than before my insulin resistance diagnosis in 2007, but I still have moments when I just want a Bismark donut. I'm not perfect. But I actively try to figure out how to satisfy my cravings minimally.

As an example: I bought a tray of fresh sushi from the grocery store. I love sushi, but it doesn't love me. I already knew artificial crab contains added sugars, so I chose a tray without that ingredient. The rice was my main nemesis. I've learned through the use of my CGM if I consume the whole tray, which is ten pieces, my sugar will spike above 250. But what if I only ate five pieces, waited an hour and then ate the other five pieces? I decided to run an experiment. I ate my five sushi pieces, savoring every bite, then set a timer for one hour. I was active outside with yardwork during that time. Then I treated myself to the second portion. Reviewing my CGM numbers later, I found this was a "green zone" way to enjoy sushi without overloading what my body can process. ("Green-zone" means to stay in target range on the CGM. My range is below 180 and above 70.)

Portion control. It really helped me.

I plan on trying the same experiment with brown rice sushi, since brown rice spikes me less than white rice.

Another trick to satisfying a craving is to buy a small size item. My bakery sells single pieces of cheesecake. The piece is too large for me to eat alone, so I share it with my husband. I also know not to eat too much of the graham cracker crust. And, because I only bought one piece, (that we finished), and not a whole cheesecake, I'm not tempted to eat more in the middle of the night. Individually packaged treats usually have nutritional content charts, too. This way you can see how many carbohydrates one serving contains.

I feel it's important to not cut out all the prior foods from our lives because of a diabetes diagnosis. This can lead to depression and binge eating–of that, I speak from experience. The notion of, "I can't eat that anymore," may create a feedback loop, causing you to eventually give in or binge that type of food. Small packages and portion control are my way of satisfying cravings, and I was able to confirm my choices were good through the use of my CGM. Prior to wearing a CGM, I had to wait until my next office visit to see if recent changes to eating patterns or habits were effectual. I prefer real-time results.

I want to circle back to potluck dinners. I've struggled to reign in my self-control and continue with healthy eating when I'm faced with a huge spread of food. Like the two potluck dinners with our families in the fall of 2021—being surrounded by loved ones and food seemed to be a caustic situation for my healthy eating habits.

Since then, I made the decision to take responsibility for my personal choices. I don't need to feel pressured to taste everyone's dish. Perhaps when the situation arises again, I'll fill up on my healthy food before I go to dinner. Or maybe I'll communicate with the family about my restrictions and that I'll be bringing a low-carb dish.

Sugar is everywhere!

Part of healthy eating is watching out for added sugar in foods. The sushi I mentioned came with a packet of soy sauce that contained high-fructose corn syrup. Instead, I used my own soy sauce that does not contain added sugar. Look at the ingredients of the foods you eat, watch out for these sneaky additions in all forms. Some examples include:

- high-fructose corn syrup
- brown sugar
- cane juice
- corn syrup

- dextrose
- fructose
- fruit nectars
- glucose
- honey
- lactose
- malt syrup
- maltose
- maple syrup
- molasses
- raw sugar
- sucrose

Keeping an eye out for these ingredients will help you manage your diabetes more effectively. I mean, why would soy sauce have sugar anyway? It's supposed to be salty. In the past, I wouldn't have looked at the ingredient list, but I do that now. I recommend you do the same. Check the ingredients of everything you eat.

Breads can have added sugar, too, which as a wheat-based carbohydrate, will spike blood sugar on its own. Read the ingredient list on the package.

If you reduce or eliminate the extra sugars from your diet, then when moments arise where you can't avoid them you won't have to worry too much. It's a percentage game. Just like keeping your sugar in the green zone most of the time allows for brief moments outside the zone.

Keep healthy snacks at the ready. You don't want to be caught off guard, unprepared when faced with an empty stomach. I try to always have a low sugar protein bar in my purse. They have protein along with the healthy carbs to help me regulate my sugars and avoid a dip—or the temptation to purchase not-so-healthy food. Also, I recommend you designate a cupboard or space in your kitchen for your diabetic food needs. That way, when you have a craving, look in your cupboard first for something to get you through.

In the past, I've frequented fast food establishments. That's a sophisticated way of saying I caved into the aroma of burgers and fries as I walked across the parking lot to my car after my shift. Grabbing a little something quick to eat seemed appealing at the time. However, using a CGM helped me realize just how bad fast food is for my body and I've now nearly eliminated all fast food from my diet. Not completely, but nearly.

I suspect there are a lot of hidden sugars in fast food. The ingredients are certainly highly processed, so my body doesn't need to work so hard to get the carbs into my bloodstream. I mean, I can grill a burger at home and fry my own potatoes and my sugar won't spike as much as if I order fast food burgers and fries. Something is very different with their ingredients compared to mine. Unfortunately, fast food is, well, fast. Home-cooked is not.

Diabetic Distress

This is a very real complication of changing everything about your eating habits, especially if your previous foods were all unhealthy. The new diabetes-friendly diet may be so incredibly foreign to you and contain foods that you've shied away from most of your life—but are now expected to eat regularly—that you may feel irritated, grumpy, depressed, frustrated, and hopeless.

The mental distress of these changes is not just "all in your head." It is very real. Please don't ignore these feelings. They are your brain's way of telling you it's not happy with all the changes you're making, and the feelings are perfectly natural.

But fear not, there are ways to avoid diabetic distress, some of which I've already mentioned, like how to deal with cravings, portion control, and learning about what works best for you within the changes you decide to make.

Prepare ahead. One way that helped me avoid diabetic distress was to prepare ahead. Utilize leftovers for lunch the next day by packing them in small containers after your meal. On my way out the door, I can easily grab the ready-to-go meal from the night before versus taking the time to find a small container with a lid that fits and scooping out a portion, all while knowing I'm running late. If I haven't prepared, I tend to purchase something at work for lunch and that's where I consume the not-so-healthy foods. I work in a grocery store pharmacy, and you might think that would be convenient to buy lunch on the days I didn't pack one, but no. Grab and go food items are expensive and will raise my blood sugar.

Other ways to prepare meals ahead so they'll be easier and less distressful include purchasing prepackaged containers of fruit, vegetables, or frozen dinners that fit your dietary needs. On my days off, I'll stock up my cupboard with protein bars, trail mix, and find the containers and lids I'll need for the coming week. I'll purchase cheese sticks, yogurt, salad ingredients, etc., to make preparing lunches all that much easier.

Preparing ahead helps me prevent uncontrollable situations.

Avoid temptation. For example: As I mentioned, I currently work in a grocery store pharmacy. Every day I walk into an environment that smells of fresh donuts, fried chicken, and hot coffee—all heavenly aromas, in my opinion. Sure, I can eat and drink all these things, but they each affect my blood sugar differently. Instead, I avoid temptation and thus reduce my diabetic distress by choosing to walk down aisles on my way to the pharmacy that don't contain food items. On most days, I've packed my lunch and snacks, so I'm not forced to shop in the store, which may lead to purchasing something less healthy for me.

Buy in bulk. Healthy eating can also be achieved by buying in bulk. When I buy a big bag of trail mix, I weigh out/ estimate one ounce/single servings and place them in snack size Ziploc bags to make snacking even easier. This way I know approximately how many carbohydrates and protein grams I'm getting, and I reduce the chances of mindless eating from the big bag. Plus, these premeasured bags are great to grab and go.

If you have a store nearby that sells food from big bins, like a bulk foods section, I have found this is a great way to try different ingredients. For example, I wanted to try steel cut oats to see what they would do to my glucose levels. Down the cereal aisle, the smallest bag had maybe two cups of oats inside, with a steep price. What if I didn't like them? What if my sugar spiked too high? Would I just throw out the remaining oats? I don't like throwing out food. So, I went to the bulk section of the store and found the same steel cut oats. I measured out a cup and placed it in a small bag with an identifying label. Not only did it save me in food waste if I didn't like them, but it also cost less than one-fourth of the packaged option down the aisle. (Steel-cut oats registered in the green zone when I only consumed 1/3 cup cooked. That seems like a small amount, but it is quite filling. I toss in a few blueberries and a splash of milk.) Now that I know I like these oats, I'll buy them in bulk because they're cheaper.

Reduce diabetic distress with a CGM. The way a continuous glucose monitor can help you reduce distress is by helping you find the foods and their portion sizes for your individual needs. Here's a sampling of what I've found for myself. I found that I can eat barley and beef soup and not spike. The same with whole wheat pasta, in moderation. I avoid white rice, but I can eat small portions of brown rice. Breads are generally going to spike my sugar, with the exception of breads containing seeds and nuts *and* with accompanying protein like peanut butter or meat and cheese. Chocolate is not as bad as I thought, in small amounts. Candy bars with nuts in bite-size portions are nice glucose bumps when I'm dipping but not able to eat a meal. A measured amount of trail mix (the trail mix I mentioned earlier) with chocolate candy bits and peanuts is a surprisingly decent snack without a spike for me. If there are dehydrated fruits, like raisins, then not so much. Charting my CGM results following these foods has helped me fashion my personal eating habits to suit my needs.

Healthy eating with diabetes or pre-diabetes can feel daunting at first, but as you move forward, step by step, you'll find the foods that you like and that keep your glucose levels in the green zone.

CHAPTER 4: TOOLBOX ESSENTIAL – CONTINUOUS GLUCOSE MONITORS

If the #1 toolbox necessity for managing my blood glucose is monitoring the foods I eat, then #2 is monitoring what those foods do to my glucose levels.

Glucometers with accompanying glucose test strips test the glucose level at that moment, which is great if you need to know exactly where your sugar level is at present. However, it's a snapshot, or like reading one page out of a novel. You're getting limited knowledge. Alternatively, if you want to see the "whole story" of where your sugar levels peaked and dipped over the course of the day, I suggest requesting a continuous glucose monitoring system from your doctor.

The following information will help you determine if using a CGM is right for you. Additionally, I'll go over the purchasing end of things, like cost, copays, and coupons.

Who would benefit from using a CGM?

Let's talk about who would benefit from using a continuous glucose monitor. They include patients suffering from glucose management issues who:

- don't like to do fingersticks regularly.
- want to learn what the foods they eat are doing to their glucose levels in real time.
- are beginning a new medication.
- want to take charge of their health now instead of later.

I feel strongly that if you've been diagnosed with blood sugar issues, you should consider trying a continuous glucose monitor for at least two weeks to get a window into what's happening in your body with the foods you eat. Every body is unique. Your body is different from another patient who also has a high A1c. Your medication treatment plan is different. You may be more sensitive to the insulin in your body than other people with the same A1c. There is no definitive chart or graph that reflects everyone all at once. The blood fasting and A1c numbers are a fixed chart, but how each body responds and *why* those numbers are where they are can be different.

Wearing a CGM gives you your unique, continual numbers and in doing so, the power to help make informed decisions about what foods you choose to eat.

Before I learned about CGMs, a friend of mine who had started a new diabetic medication would often get so sick she'd have to go home early from her job or call out altogether. No doubt, there can be some pretty hefty side effects with some diabetic medications, but I do wonder if some of her symptoms were due to low blood sugar because the medication was working "too well." If she had been wearing a CGM, she could have had some additional metrics to help her understand if her feelings of illness were due to other factors. Of course, she could have also poked her finger and tested her blood for a snapshot, but she had a difficult time with that type of blood test.

I do want to point out that my friend's diabetes and the steps taken to manage it interfered with her ability to perform her job. She had some sick pay banked to cover her absent days and missed hours, but at some point, that ran out. (I guess we should add lost wages and the possibility of being an unreliable employee to the list of complications of diabetes.)

Everyone responds differently to medications and can sometimes cause your body to react in odd ways as it's adjusting. By using a CGM, you can learn earlier if you are not adapting, which may help to limit or avoid some of the negative side effects from these lifestyle/treatment implementations.

At this point in time, CGMs are relatively new in the diabetes landscape. My grandmother never had the opportunity to use one. She was meticulous in monitoring her sugars with finger-pokes, yet she eventually developed renal failure, and she passed away at age seventy-five. Three quarters of a century is a long time to live, no doubt, which is probably longer than her predecessors who had diabetes. At present, my mother has outlived her mother by nearly five years, which is a testament to the advancements in diabetes care in the last thirty years.

Now, with new technology like CGMs and medications, who knows how much longer a patient can live with diabetes? But I don't want to simply live longer, I want to be able to ***live better***, to have mobility and energy to do the things I love. I do see how my own sugar battle is improved by wearing a CGM. If I keep my sugars in the green zone as much as possible, I will avoid potential complications that could lead to less years living. But I can also ensure those extra years have less diabetic-related issues.

Another example of who might consider wearing a CGM. Older, long-running diabetics might want to consider asking their doctor about CGM systems. My seventy-nine-year-old mother, who initially scoffed at my CGM, finally got set up with one. She uses an insulin pump and has for several years, but she still must know how much insulin to dispense. She thought she had figured out a good formula for counting the carbs she ate, doing the math in her head, and calculating the insulin dose. Unfortunately, this didn't work in the long run.

She gave me permission to share her numbers with you. Her A1c was 10.6% when she started wearing her CGM. After three months of seeing her blood sugars in real time compared to the foods she was eating, then altering or reducing carb intake, and adjusting insulin doses, her A1c dropped remarkably to 7.4%. Her doctors were beyond flabbergasted. Three months later, her A1c dropped further to 6.9%. Through diet and proper insulin dosing in her insulin pump, she is seeing numbers she hasn't seen in decades. Imagine if she could have had this technology years ago. Think of all the fingersticks she could have avoided!

My mother has told me that by being able to see the CGM numbers on the graph associated with the foods she eats, she has been able to predict what certain carb-loaded foods will do to her blood sugar. Therefore, she now avoids those foods or limits them to smaller amounts. That's how she's been able to reduce her A1c—by using the CGM readings to guide her in real time to make better eating decisions. And by reducing the number of carbohydrates she eats, she also reduces the amount of insulin needed to process those carbs. It's a win-win situation.

To recap, insulin users can benefit from wearing a CGM both by being able to make better food choices and by being able to dial in their insulin dosage better.

Instant Accountability

A huge benefit of wearing a CGM is the instant accountability it brings me after consuming less-healthy food choices. This accountability comes in the form of an alarm alerting me to glucose levels outside of the green zone, high or low. If I have my high alarm turned off, I can still see my spike, but the instant accountability isn't as strong in my opinion. I'll go over the alarm settings more in chapter fifteen.

Here's an example. I was craving a Bismark, like I do, so I thought I'd visit the new bake shop in the neighborhood. Not being able to decide from the many options, I loaded a dozen different delicacies and totted them off to work, thinking my coworkers might enjoy a treat, too. I turned off my CGM's upper alarm, feeling confident I could pace myself with portion control to keep my numbers in the green zone. I was mistaken, however. I quickly consumed a whole portion and then watched my CGM silently spike out of the stratosphere over the next hour. I drank a lot of water in a panic with the hopes of diluting my blood levels, and I ate a protein bar. It seemed like forever for my sugar level to come back down. But eventually it did.

Later, for round two, I ate a protein bar first, drank a glass of water, then ate only half of a Bismark. This time my numbers stayed in the green zone.

What I learned about my body is sweet carbohydrates on an empty stomach are bad, bad, bad. If I wait to eat a smaller amount of the same treat until after I've eaten some protein and water, my body will handle it better.

I also learned that I respond better to hearing my alarm remind me I overindulged. I shouldn't have turned off my upper alarm on the day of the Bismarcks. I should have let it blare away. Perhaps I wouldn't have eaten an entire serving if I knew the alarm would shrill. I don't know. What I do know is I felt sneaky, thinking I was pulling one over my CGM. But really all I was doing was hurting my own body and my future health. I need the alarms to keep me on track, embarrassing or not.

So, the instant accountability that can be achieved when using a CGM is dependent on the user. If I use my device as a training tool in my arsenal of diabetes management, I can determine how much of a particular food I can eat. I can also determine the order in which I eat foods and how that *does* make a difference in my body. Your body may be different than mine, so keep that in mind.

It will be a long time before I buy another Bismark, and when I do, I will know how much of it I can eat, what other options to eat or drink first, and if I need to space out portions throughout the day to avoid large spikes.

Learn to recognize what you feel when your number is high or low.

One of the best outcomes of wearing a CGM is learning to recognize what your body feels like with sugar highs and lows. Sugar highs are deceiving to say the least. Most people don't recognize the feelings they feel when their sugar levels are high. I didn't know my body felt a certain way when my sugar was elevated. That's another reason why diabetes is often referred to as a silent killer. What I discovered was the different kinds of yuckiness I felt throughout the day were associated with what was happening with my sugar.

Here's what I feel: High sugar, or a reading above 180, makes me feel nauseous and my heart races. I may break out in a slight sweat. Falling sugar makes me yawn repeatedly. Low sugar makes me feel a little flushed, confused, and my brain glitches. I also get nauseous but it's slightly different than the high sugar nauseousness. Sometimes my tongue will tingle, or I'll get the shakes. So, basically, when I can't say the words I'm trying to say and my hands are shaking, I know I need to eat immediately. It doesn't matter if my low alarm hasn't gone off yet. I've learned to listen to my body and prevent a deep low. I get out in front of the sugar rollercoaster and slow the descent with smart food choices that won't quickly spike my blood. If I wait too long and the alarm goes off, then I need to eat some simple glucose to quickly pull my sugar up and get my brain working again. But I have to be careful not to overdo it or else I'll bring on another sugar crash.

Because I've paid attention to what my body feels like during extreme low glucose levels, I've been able to go without my CGM for a week or so and still maintain good numbers. I've learned what certain foods and portion sizes will do to my sugar levels, so I know fairly well what my number would look like even in the absence of a CGM. The only problem is sometimes my medication pushes my numbers lower than my logbook results, and for that reason, I try to always wear my CGM. Additionally, I keep my blood glucometer nearby as a backup to stay on top of my sugar readings.

Again, wearing the CGM has made it possible for me to discern what *my* body feels like during the different stages of blood sugar cycles. Your body's response may be different than mine, so keep that in mind.

What about a person who doesn't have blood sugar problems? Can they wear a CGM?

Prescription CGMs are intended for diabetics using insulin, pre-diabetic patients, and those who suffer from hypoglycemia. If a patient does not fit these qualifications but still wants to wear a CGM, they can investigate other non-pharmaceutical options. A quick internet search will bring up companies that are jumping into the CGM market outside of diabetic needs.

Author note: Since completion of this book, Dexcom announced that coming in the summer of 2024, they will release an over-the-counter CGM available for non-insulin patients to purchase without a prescription. Abbott has already released an OTC version in the UK, available without a prescription.

Something to be aware of for non-diabetics concerning CGM readings. The glucose readings might be low. CGM readings are more reliable when measuring high sugar than when measuring low numbers. Someone may falsely be led to believe they have hypoglycemia because of wearing a CGM. So, it would be wise for the non-diabetic to also purchase a glucometer and double check the low CGM readings against the actual fingerstick readings. Even diabetics wearing a CGM are prompted to also check their blood sugar when the numbers show too low.

Personally, I feel non-qualifying people (non-diabetics or non-glucose challenged) wanting to wear a CGM should purchase from outside companies that are not catering to the diabetic/hypoglycemic insurance-covered pharmaceutical crowd. I say this from a pharmacy technician's point of view. If everyone decided to try out a CGM—and could get their doctor to write a prescription—there would be an instant shortage of CGMs.

My doctor brother pointed out that medical professionals are held to a standard of only writing scripts for drugs or devices that are medically needed. *(Here's a pharmacy tech nugget: Have you ever had a prescription delayed due to a "prior authorization" or p.a.? That's your health insurance wanting your doctor to explain why they thought you needed the prescription. The doctor must explain and justify their decision with the insurance. This happens all the time with many different medications, and yes, with CGMs, too.)*

Will health insurance cover the cost of a CGM?

Not all insurances will extend coverage even if you are a qualifying patient. You can find out easily if your insurance will cover a continuous glucose monitor simply by calling the phone number on the back of your insurance card and asking. Most insurances have websites listing approved medications and devices, so you could also check there.

I recommend you first find out if your insurance will cover a device, get the details like brand and model, then ask your doctor for a prescription. Some doctors won't prescribe a CGM (even if you are a qualifying patient) because they assume your insurance won't cover it, and they don't want to deal with a prior authorization. So, I suggest going in armed with knowledge and let your doctor know exactly what your insurance will cover.

Remember, a prescription is needed to purchase a CGM from a pharmacy. If your doctor is hesitant to prescribe one, it could simply be because of the prior authorization hassle I mentioned earlier. Knowing ahead of your doctor's visit whether you are covered by insurance will help immensely.

Alternatively, if you find your insurance doesn't offer coverage, even though you qualify, you can still get a prescription for a CGM from your doctor and then pay cash at the pharmacy. There is no need to pay the full retail price, however. I suggest checking GoodRx.com and other discount drug companies for the best price location to fill your prescription and provide the discount coupon to that pharmacy. One two-week FreeStyle Libre3 sensor with a GoodRx coupon runs around $75.

Before you pay any cash, always check the manufacturer's website for a one-time free-trial coupon. I've seen those used with FreeStyle Libre purchases as a pharmacy technician. There are some caveats, however, so read the fine print. I noticed on FreeStylelibre.com they have a phone number to call for possible reduction of cost for insured patients.

Dexcom.com also has information that can be accessed about insurance coverage.

Both websites are loaded with information and helpful tidbits to navigate the world of continuous glucose monitoring.

Another option if your insurance doesn't cover CGMs is to make your purchase through one of the new companies springing up on the internet. The ones I have seen are on a subscription basis. The quality and accuracy of these other companies' products are unknown to me. Do your research and buyer beware.

A patient recently came in and reported that their doctor had free samples of FreeStyle Libre in their office. The patient had been set up, having the doctor apply the first sensor to their arm, and were dropping off a script for refills.

So, there's one more option. Ask your doctor if they have free samples.

What will you gain from trying a CGM?

You might be wondering after reading about the insurance coverage or non-coverage, is it worth the effort to try a CGM? *What's in it for me?*

You'll gain knowledge of what your fasting blood sugar numbers are for 14 days in a row. You'll be able to see in real time what the foods you eat on a regular basis are doing to your sugar levels. Foods you thought were fine might not be. Foods you thought were bad might not be as bad. You could gain valuable insight into your lifestyle and how your activity affects your blood sugar levels, helping you to see the benefit of physical activity. All this data could then be used to make subtle changes to benefit your overall health. If nothing else, this data may be used to help you keep future medical expenses to a minimum, such as extra doctor's appointments or medication costs.

If you've decided to pursue a CGM at this point, great! I wish you the best with adding this device to your toolbox for managing blood sugar levels.

CHAPTER 5: TOOLBOX ESSENTIAL – LOGBOOK

Logbook

I'm more of a physical person than a digital person. For example, I do better if I can hold a book in my hands versus using an electronic device. (*Which is ironic because most of the sales I've made on my fiction books were from ebooks, not paperbacks.*) If you also like physical books, then I recommend getting a logbook to track your numbers, foods, and other health related stats.

Some CGMs also offer a digital notes option within the app, but I found that to be limiting for the notes I wanted to take. But that's just me. Maybe digital is your thing.

Either way, keeping track of what you eat can help to properly interpret the results.

My first Libre was the "14-day" model. The readings would sometimes be 10-20 points off of my fingerstick readings, so I took that into account when reviewing. What I found to be the biggest help was seeing the sharp climb after consuming carbs. I began experimenting with different foods to get a reading on what my regular, day-to-day foods were doing to my sugar levels. How many points did that banana make my sugar climb? I'd note the number before eating the banana, then watch over the next two hours to see what my body did with it and note those numbers. An example would be beginning at number 90, the peak number 140, then a drop or bottom out to 95 after two hours. The banana raised me 50 points on its own. I can notate these findings in my logbook and try again another time, referencing this example.

Author note: An update on the banana experiment: ripe bananas, or those that are deep yellow with browning skins, spike my sugars more compared to a firm banana that still has hints of green on the ends. One-half of a ripe banana will raise me 50 points, whereas it takes a whole firm banana to do the same. Interesting. This experiment definitely went in the logbook!

When performing these kinds of food experiments, if my sugar level shoots out of my green zone, then whatever food I ate comes under scrutiny. Did I eat too big of a portion? Did the foods have added sugars I wasn't aware of? Did I eat too many different forms of carbohydrates, i.e.: hamburger (bun) and fries?

Of course, these kinds of experiments can be done with glucose test strips, too, in snapshot fashion, but you'll need three to four strips. If you were given a prescription for glucose test strips, you probably have a daily allotment and insurance won't cover additional strips early. So, these kinds of tests may require that you purchase your own test strips to use at your own discretion. Just keep that in mind.

The point here is to think about writing down in a logbook (or notating in your CGM app) your findings to assist in monitoring your progress.

Libreview (for use with FreeStyle Libre products)

Whether you use the FreeStyle Libre app on your cell phone as the reader, or if you use the FreeStyle branded reader device, **Libreview.com** will retain your reader's records privately and securely but only if you upload them. The FreeStyle Libre2 reader device will retain readings for only a few months due to the small onboard memory, so don't rely on the reader to hold all your past numbers. I made that mistake and now I don't have reports for a large part of 2022. I have my A1c blood tests and fasting glucose numbers from my healthcare visits, and my own recollection that I held steady for that year, but I wish I would have uploaded my reader's data to Libreview.

That being said, Libreview seems to only hold onto data for two years, so the best way to save your records is to download the printable reports in PDF version from Libreview. I use the 90-day setting. After downloading, I go into my phone's calendar and make a note 90 days out to get my reports again off Libreview.

Another feature with Libreview is you can digitally share your data with your doctor. A special login on the doctor's end gives them secure access to your data. I haven't done this yet with my PA, but it's on my list of things to try.

To upload your reader's data, connect the USB cord that comes with the reader to your computer and follow the instructions on Libreview.com. If using your cell phone as your reader, log into Libreview and follow the instructions. I use the FreeStyle Libre3 app on my phone, and once I log into Libreview, my data instantly displays.

CHAPTER 6: TOOLBOX ESSENTIALS – DOCTOR VISITS, BLOODWORK, AND TESTS

I haven't always gone to the doctor on a regular basis in the past, but I'm a big proponent of regular visits now. They really help me stay on track with my diabetes.

Managing my diabetes is a team effort with my healthcare provider. At my visits with my PA, we go over recent bloodwork and evaluate my progress and medication effectiveness. If I bring my printed ninety-day report from Libreview, she can see my weekly averages and number of hypoglycemic episodes along with the patterns brought on by my eating routines. And because I also used a logbook, I can match up meals to the printed data from Libreview.

Something my data revealed was that my sugar level throughout the night would dip down to 80, then around 6:00 a.m. would start to climb upward to about 124 without food consumption—which would be the time in the morning I'd test for fasting blood sugar levels. So, my fasting glucose numbers were coming in high. Not everyone's body does this, but because of wearing the CGM, I was able to see that my body does.

This is called the "Dawn Phenomenon." My body's glucagon activates in the wee hours of the morning and tells the liver to release some stored glucose to wake me up. I first noticed this when I was on the Keto diet and my fasting glucose levels were high even though my A1c was good. (Remember, this was the point in time when I started using a glucometer, so I don't know how long my morning sugars had been coming in high.) I researched online and read about the Dawn Phenomenon and discussed it with my PA.

What exactly is the A1c test and why does it matter?

I want to touch on this because even though I understood the A1c numbers and what constituted a normal or abnormal range, I didn't know the significance of the A1c test. Upon asking around with my coworkers, family and friends, I realized most people don't understand what the A1c number means either (i.e. a certain range tells you if you're diabetic or not.) So, I dug a little deeper and I learned even more as I researched this book. Here's my simplified, bare bones explanation.

Red blood cells contain a protein called hemoglobin which transports oxygen from the lungs to the cells, then picks up carbon dioxide and delivers it to the lungs to be expelled from the body. The cycle begins again with a new pick-up of oxygen for transfer. Think of hemoglobin as a taxi on a looping track. New red blood cells are constantly entering the bloodstream after being created in the bone marrow.

Our red blood cells have a lifespan of around three to four months. During that time, we eat carbohydrates that are converted to glucose which floats in the bloodstream, ready to be put to work, ready to be helped into the cells or otherwise utilized by the body. If there is excess glucose in our blood than what our body is able to utilize, it can stick to the hemoglobin taxis like a barnacle on the side of a ship. The glucose does not drop off, nor is it transferred into the cells once it attaches to the hemoglobin; it just hangs on until the cell dies.

The older the cell, the more glucose barnacles have possibly attached. Therefore, when a drop of blood is analyzed for an A1c test, the older blood cells tattletale on you in the form of a percentage. What percentage of your hemoglobin is covered with glucose barnacles? You might have told your doctor that you followed your diet plan religiously and kept your blood sugar in good ranges, but your hemoglobin says, "Nuh uh, oh no you didn't."

Author note: Free-floating sugar in the blood is measured by glucometers. Glucose stuck to the hemoglobin is measured by the A1c test.

It is normal for some glucose to stick to hemoglobin. But once the amount reaches 5.7%, the hemoglobin's ability to effectively transfer oxygen and carbon dioxide is diminished. The higher the A1c reading, the less oxygen transfer that is taking place.[2] Oxygen must wait for another taxi to come along, one that is younger and hasn't lived long enough to be covered in glucose. When your red blood cell dies, the glucose is broken down and eliminated from the body.

Why is it a big deal if oxygen has to wait for another taxi? Well, for example, oxygen is needed throughout the body for energy, healing, or thinking. Reduction in these levels can create difficulty in these other types of areas, which creates alternate side effects. Without proper oxygen transfer, muscle exhaustion comes earlier, and wounds heal slower, among other things.

Can someone live with a high A1c and diminished oxygen in their cells? Of course. It happens all the time. I'll overhear people talking about their test results and how their A1c was 12%, or 11%, or 10%. That's much higher than my highest level at 6.8%. But damage from reduced oxygen accumulates over time, slowly building in the system. Staying at such high levels increases the likelihood of these issues manifesting.

Now consider that because the cell lifespan of four months is so short, a drastic change to eating habits, even in just a few months, can lower the A1c count, like with my mother, and myself. Blood cells born today, brand new shiny taxi cabs, can be kept pristine if the amount of glucose floating in the bloodstream is kept at a good level.

In knowing that I'm keeping my little oxygen taxis in good working order, I know I'm allowing my body the resources it needs to operate, heal, and thrive. In the study I referenced above [2], they found that participants who were prediabetic and screen diagnosed diabetic (those who previously didn't know they had a high A1c until participating in the study) had lower oxygen levels than non-diabetics, poor kidney filtration numbers, higher cholesterol values, and more. This was an unintended revelation that prediabetes stage (A1c 5.7%-6.4%) brings damage to our bodies.

Additionally, the A1c test is an indicator that too much glucose is staying in the bloodstream where it can cause damage. This is usually caused by the cells not accepting the floating glucose by way of insulin, known as insulin resistance. High A1c numbers indicate the level of malfunction between the insulin and cells, and this is where a patient is diagnosed with diabetes. If the patient is eating an overabundance of carbohydrates, the body simply cannot process and utilize all the sugar. Some will get stored as fat. Some will be eliminated. Some will stick to the hemoglobin. And on and on. Exercise can help use up excess glucose and eating less carbohydrates lessens the strain on the body to process as much, too. Some people will always be able to handle the glucose in their bloodstream. Others, like me, struggle for whatever reason, be it genetics or improperly functioning organs or just because my body has a harder time processing sugar.

Keep this in mind if you struggle. Learning about your body and how it reacts may help lessen the burden for you.

Who else should consider taking an A1c test?

You've been tested and you know your result, and now you know the significance of the A1c, and you want to shout it from the rooftops to raise awareness that everyone should get their A1c checked, too . . . oh, wait, that might just be me. When I first found out I had an elevated A1c, probably due to genetics and my misunderstanding of carbohydrates, I immediately thought of my siblings. I wanted them to get checked, too. I wanted them to become aware of what might be happening inside their bodies so they could take measures to halt any potential damage. My thoughts were all meant well, but I found when I shared those thoughts with my siblings, I didn't get the responses I expected.

Remember, diabetes or insulin resistance tends to run in families and doesn't always have symptoms. When a type 2 diabetes diagnosis is found in one member of a family, other blood relatives might consider being evaluated, too. A simple

A1c test will establish a baseline, a point in time with an associated number. However, this is easier said than done. Encouraging blood relatives to get their A1c checked can be frustrating, especially when they are not receptive to your reasoning. I speak from experience.

I tried to get my sister to get her A1c tested once I discovered mine was already 5.9%. She is five years younger than me and at that time she was around thirty-two years old. I told her that if I could go back five years and see where I was, I would do it. She responded with, "Yeah, I need to get that done." Sadly, she didn't get her blood tested until she was forty-five, following a bout of pneumonia that hospitalized her for a week. When she viewed her lab work later on, she saw her fasting blood sugar while in the hospital was over 200. She asked her doctor if she could be diabetic and if he would give her an A1c test. At first, he declined, stating something along the line that when we're sick, our blood sugar does some wonky things, and not to worry about it. I had pestered my sister many times over the years about getting the test, so she finally persisted and asked the doctor to at least just do the test so she could get a baseline, since her mother and sister were both diabetic. The test was run, and her A1c came back as 6.8%.

Diabetic.

The doctor was baffled.

My sister was upset.

You can probably imagine why.

Another sister, the one who my mother suspected was having hypoglycemia episodes as a child, is ten years younger than me. She acted upon our insistence to get tested, and at age 42, she learned she was insulin resistant. She has since lowered her numbers to 5.7% with diet alone. Great job!

As in the case of sister #1, some doctors are hesitant to administer the test, thinking it's not necessary. Additionally, some doctor's offices are booked out for many weeks, discouraging anyone wanting to get their blood tested promptly. There are always the at-home test options, which are available for purchase online and at many pharmacies. Also, medical laboratories like Quest Labs will perform patient-ordered tests, too, for a reasonable cost.

Getting an A1c test is easier than ever. The sooner a patient can learn if their body is struggling to manage blood glucose levels, the better. However, sometimes encouraging others to get tested and providing information about how to go about doing it is all you can do.

Set up access to My Chart or Patient Portal

Whether you implement continuous glucose monitoring into your toolbox of diabetic management or not, I recommend you set up your My Chart or Patient Portal with your care provider, if you haven't already. All too often when I speak with family or friends about their health or recent doctor visits, I'll bring up the question, "Does your doctor's office have a 'my chart' service for patients?" or "Have you looked at your 'my chart'?" Their response is, "What's that?" or "I don't know."

Using My Chart, you can send messages directly to your doctor or their medical staff with questions or requests. This has proven for me to be the better option to communicate with my provider versus calling the office, which usually results in leaving a voice mail. Medical phone tag stinks due to HIPAA. If you miss their return call, they can't leave a detailed message on voice mail, so you'll have to call again and pray you don't end up in the voice mail loop. But with the My Chart option, the doctor can respond to your question in detail, and you can read the response on your own time. No phone tag.

Similarly, if you have lab work done outside the office, like with LabCorp, Quest, etc., get yourself signed up and logged in. These types of lab services usually have tracking graphs that allow you to see at a glance what your previous numbers were and if you've improved or not. Very helpful when taking charge of your own health . . . or writing a book.

CHAPTER 7: TOOLBOX ESSENTIAL - MEDICATIONS

Miracle Pills

As a pharmacy technician, I am privy to the confidential medical advice my pharmacist offers patients during consultation. I've noticed some generalities among patients that, without revealing any protected health information, I'd like to point out as they relate to treatment of diabetes and diabetes complications.

Generally speaking, people -

- don't want to die/or be in pain.
- don't like change.
- put too much reliance on the medication they are taking be it for diabetes, cholesterol, or heart problems, etc., and not enough emphasis on themselves to alter their diet to assist the performance of the medication.

I personally relate to all three of these findings. For me and my husband, we both had to make big changes when he had his heart attack—because he didn't want to die at age forty-four. I didn't want him to die, either. That should go without saying, but I'll say it anyway.

Then I found out about my own health issues soon after. Together, we made enormous changes to our diets, and for a while, we stuck to those changes. Then, over time, we slacked off, little by little, because permanent change requires continual effort. And then, I found myself relying on my medication to do all the work. That felt so much easier than being proactive with my health.

I see this all the time in the pharmacy, too. Patients don't want to be in pain. They don't want to die, yet they don't seem to want it bad enough to adhere to permanent changes.

I know it's hard. I've dealt with falling off the wagon, too. But the trick is to get back up, dust off, then jump back on the wagon.

Modern medicine is pretty awesome in what it can do to help the body, but there are limits with a lot of medications, and the patient has to do their part. Simply taking a pill, or drinking a solution, doesn't always fix the problem. We have to do our part for our medications to be the most effective.

Adherence

An entirely different matter is lack of adherence to the medication. I'm guilty of this, too. Some of my medications are on auto-refill and are ready to pick up before my bottle at home is empty—because of all the times I didn't take my meds before bed.

Personally, I've found that when I use a daily pill container and load my medications a week at a time, I'm more likely to take them on a regular basis. If I'm tired and have to open each vial for all my meds (because the daily pill container is empty), I find I'll only open the Celebrex because of my back pain. Missing my medications can cause disruptions in what it is doing to help me, so I try to load the pill case so it's easier not to forget or ignore taking them.

Do you struggle with medication adherence, too? You are not alone. But with reminders or pill containers or alarms, you can lessen the burden.

Pharmacy tech nugget: When pharmaceutical companies perform studies and tests on drugs, the subjects take the drug (or placebo) every day. The results of the studies are based on taking the medication as directed, not when the patient feels like it. To get the full benefit of my medication, I must take it as directed.

CHAPTER 8: TOOLBOX ESSENTIAL - GLUCOMETER (AT-HOME FINGERSTICK)

Glucometer

If you are newly diagnosed diabetic, you will most likely be prescribed a glucometer (fingerstick kit) along with the test strips, lancets, and lancing device. Learning how to check your current blood sugar numbers and how to decipher the reading will be important steps.

If your doctor did not prescribe you a kit, no worries. You don't need a prescription to buy one for yourself. Finger-stick kits are inexpensive. It's the test strips that can cost a lot, so shop wisely. Here in my neck of the woods at my local chain pharmacy, True Metrix is an affordable brand. Their strips are rather inexpensive and are available in lower cost packages for cash-paying customers.

For newly diagnosed insulin resistant or pre-diabetes patients, I encourage you to buy your own kit. Try checking your fasting blood glucose every morning for a week to see where your body levels out after no food for eight hours. The results can be instrumental and inspiring throughout the day when it comes to food choices. Remember, normal fasting glucose range is under 100.

Another reason I recommend having your own blood glucose testing kit is to be able to double check the accuracy of a continuous glucose monitor. CGMs are not perfect and should only be viewed as one tool in the overall management of diabetes. Sometimes, for whatever reason, my CGM will show a low glucose reading that I doubt. If I'm in a situation where I can wait it out—wait and watch for my CGM to correct itself—I'll do that. However, If I'm at work or know I will be driving soon, I will check my blood with my glucometer to put my mind at ease. At work, in a high-paced pharmacy, I don't want my mind to become fuzzy while I wait out my CGM. I need to know if I should take a glucose tab. I used to just pop a tab out of an abundance of caution, but then after learning how to read the CGM results better, I found I didn't always have to supplement with glucose tabs. Granted, sometimes I can feel the hypo moment coming on before the alarm goes off and, in that case, it's a no brainer.

I also suggest not to wait to get a glucose kit of your own, like I did. They are compact and easy to store. In fact, you can put one in your purse or backpack, so you always have it with you. You can keep a kit at your place of work and one at home, if you don't have a way of carrying one with you. However, don't leave your glucometer and strips in the car. High temperatures can damage the sensitive equipment.

Tips for the fingerstick

Wash your hands with soap and warm water to clean off excess dirt and grime. Some moisturizing soaps contain sugar-based humectants that can alter your blood sugar reading, so use a simple mild soap or even dish soap and warm water to clean your hands before testing. Air dry or use a clean paper towel to dry.

In the event you do not have access to soap and water, hand sanitizer or an alcohol swab can be used to clean the finger. Be sure to let the moisture dry completely before testing to minimize the chance for an altered reading.

Use the lancing device to draw blood (after loading a new lancet into the device), gently squeeze finger if necessary to bring out a drop of blood. Insert a test strip into the glucometer according to directions, then bring your finger with the blood drop to the exposed end of the test strip and touch gently. The strip will “suck” some of the blood into the strip and your glucometer should chime or beep to let you know an adequate sample has been achieved. Clean your finger of remaining blood and cover if necessary.

Some professionals recommend wiping the first drop of blood with gauze and testing the second drop. I’ve scoured the internet on this method only to find conflicting information. My recommendation to you would be to ask your health care provider what they recommend.

Use a sharps container or an empty milk jug to dispose of used lancets. Don’t reuse lancets as bacteria can be introduced into your body, causing infection.

CHAPTER 9: TOOLBOX ESSENTIAL – ACTIVE LIFESTYLE

Motion is Lotion

Active bodies burn more calories. True. Walking for a steady twenty to thirty minutes uses large muscle groups in the legs which in turn expends the glucose stored in the cells of those muscles. Our bodies will replace the used glucose with more glucose, thus pulling it out of the bloodstream. Remember my story of climbing the stairs to the third floor and how my blood sugar crashed? I hadn't eaten in a while, so there wasn't much sugar in my bloodstream to draw from as my muscles worked. That's why my number plummeted, and my legs turned to gelatin. But the concept was proven. Using large muscle groups brought my blood sugar down.

That example is extreme, and I didn't really understand at the time what was happening. Otherwise, I could have prepared by eating first, then expending energy. That would have been like a freebie meal in a way. Because of wearing a CGM during that example, however, I was able to see exactly what happened to my glucose when I pushed my leg muscles to exhaustion.

My personal goal is to walk at least six days a week for a solid half hour. Walking is great for clearing the mind . . . and lots of other great health benefits. Motion is lotion. My physical therapist states this mantra often. If this is difficult for you, ask your doctor about other types of exercises that will suit you and your capabilities. There are many alternatives out there.

Exercise also lowers my stress levels, clears my mind, and helps me regain focus. The stress component is a big one. I won't go into detail on that subject in this book because there is too much information to cover concerning how stress affects blood sugar levels and type 2 diabetes. If you recall in my personal history, the year I was diagnosed diabetic I started working in the pharmacy. The pandemic was in full swing, and my stress levels were off the charts. I'm sure it didn't help me in managing my sugar numbers one bit.

Needless to say, efforts to control stress will be beneficial in more ways than one.

CHAPTER 10: TOOLBOX ESSENTIAL - BLOOD PRESSURE MONITOR AND PULSE OXIMETER

With my family history of kidney failure, I'm watching my blood pressure closely. High blood pressure can damage the kidneys' ability to filter waste out of the body by weakening or narrowing the tiny vessels in the kidneys. When this happens, waste builds up in the blood, creating the need for dialysis, like with my grandmother. By having my own blood pressure machine at home, I can gather numbers outside of the doctor's office.

Other complications of high blood pressure are stroke, heart attack, heart failure, aneurysm, eye problems, memory problems, and dementia, to name a few.

Pulse oximeters are the little hinged reader that gets placed on your fingertip at the doctor's office. It reads the oxygen levels in the blood and measures your pulse. These gadgets became popular during the Covid pandemic, and our pharmacy struggled to keep them in stock. If you get one of these, make sure when you use it you are sitting down, with your hand resting in your lap or on the arm of a chair below the level of your heart. If your hand is raised, you'll get a low reading and that might make you panic. Try different fingers and even a toe to see how the numbers vary.

Author note: Having devices like these at home are nice to be able to catch medical issues earlier. However, don't rely on the readings for self-diagnosis. If the blood pressure cuff isn't on correctly, your number might be incorrect. Please don't hesitate to call 911 if there are symptoms of a heart attack or any other medical emergency.

CHAPTER 11: TOOLBOX RECAP

So, there you have it. I've shared with you my toolbox of battleplans, gadgets and devices, and medical insights that have helped me succeed moving forward as I continue my diabetic journey.

Looking back to 2007, when I learned I had a glucose balancing issue, resulting with a high A1c level, I made the dramatic change of eliminating sugared sodas from my diet which I think helped me immensely through the years. If I hadn't stopped, it's entirely likely I would have reached the diabetic threshold earlier in life than I did. And yet, I still crossed that line eventually, even with the use of medication, because sugared soda wasn't the only high carb/sugar I was ingesting.

Then I added a continuous glucose monitor to my toolbox and I learned so much about my eating habits and what was happening in my body. I firmly believe everyone who struggles with glucose management could benefit by wearing a CGM, even if it's only for two weeks, once or twice a year.

My experiences with using a CGM after so many years of struggling to keep my sugars in the green zone have inspired me enough to write this book—to pass on information to those who may not be aware of CGMs or have wondered if CGMs would benefit them.

PART C

CHAPTER 12: HOW DO C.G.M.'S WORK?

I've discussed many benefits of wearing a continuous glucose monitor and how they can help you with your food choices, resulting in better glucose numbers, but how exactly do they work?

Continuous glucose monitors have a thin filament that is inserted into the skin just far enough to reach the interstitial fluid beneath the skin layer. The filament is flexible, so a needle is needed to pierce the skin providing an open way for the filament placement. The needle then retracts into the applicator and the filament remains in place. The whole application time is like a half of a tenth of a second. It's super-fast.

The filament contains an enzyme called glucose oxidase. Through the power of this enzyme and the oxidation reaction to glucose in the fluid just under the skin's surface, the technology within the filament transmits your blood sugar level from the sensor to the reader device or cell phone.

Each CGM sensor has a limited amount of enzyme on the filament, therefore the wear time is limited (fourteen days for the Freestyle Libre products, ten days for Dexcom) before it'll need to be applied again.

If you want to learn more about the enzymatic process, try an internet search for "CGM glucose oxidase."

The sensor has an onboard battery, and most have built-in transmitters. The FreeStyle Libre3 has a transmitter and also a memory chip that will hold many hours of data. I know this because there have been times when my phone died during the night, but after I recharged and reconnected to the FreeStyle sensor, retroactive readings uploaded to my phone, filling in the graph with the missed activity.

An important thing to note about CGMs is that some substances can interfere with the glucose reading, including (but not limited to): hydroxyurea, acetaminophen, salicylic acid, tetracycline, and ascorbic acid(vitamin c).[3] I keep these factors in mind and am prepared to do a fingerstick if my numbers are questionable after taking acetaminophen or vitamin C.

Whenever I begin a new FreeStyle sensor, I get an alert stating that high doses of vitamin C can cause the readings of the CGM to be off. Currently, (2023) that's the only substance included in the warning.

The microscopic technology and scientific research behind these glucose monitors astounds me. These devices are certainly gamechangers in my battle against diabetes.

CHAPTER 13: TIPS ON APPLICATION, MAINTENANCE, REMOVAL AND MORE

Attaching a sensor

Everyone has dead skin cells and natural oils on the surface of their skin. If you decide to try out a CGM device, to get the best adhesion, you need to prepare the skin's surface properly. I've tried several methods and failed multiple times to keep the sensor in place the full two weeks. So rather than go through your own trial and error, I want to offer the methods that worked for me. If you prefer, I've also posted some short videos on YouTube demonstrating my tips and tricks of using the FreeStyle Libre3. My channel name is CGM Tips.

FreeStyle Libre instructions recommend attaching the sensor to the back side of the upper arm, where we tend to have more of a fat layer. I've often seen people with the device situated more toward the outer side of the arm. I learned from experience that it will most likely get knocked off before their two weeks completes. My biggest culprit is bumping into door jambs. Been there, done that.

The unit is more protected when placed further back on the arm.

To help visualize this, imagine your left arm hanging down, relaxed. If you look down at it from above, and use a clock face for reference, then 12:00 is the front of the left arm, 3:00 is the inside of the arm next to the body, 6:00 the backside, and 9:00 is the outside of the arm. You want your sensor to be placed somewhere between 6:00 and 8:00, and also about halfway between your elbow and shoulder. Up higher is fine. My sensor is usually visible if I wear a short-sleeved shirt. I prefer the 7:00 area.

Even with proper preparation to the skin, sometimes the sensor adhesive may begin to lift away before the complete two weeks have passed. I've often used a regular bandage to prevent further lifting and to keep the filament in place in my arm.

Once the filament pulls out from the skin, it cannot be re-inserted. The sensor is done. An error message will display on your reading device to let you know information is no longer transmitting.

Additional application tips

Based on experience, I suggest that the first time you apply a sensor, cover it with a large bandage immediately from day one. This can help your mind and body adjust to protecting the device, which you may forget you're wearing—believe me. Over time, you'll learn to protect your arm as you go through tight spaces or doorways. All it takes is one sensor being flicked off by accident to make you hyperaware of the situation.

I suggest applying the sensor in the morning hours. This will give your arm time to heal from the insertion. I've attached sensors in the evening hours and found I struggled sleeping because my arm felt sore. Now I only attach in the morning.

Apply to clean, dry skin, and keep it that way for twenty-four hours. I don't shower right before or after applying a sensor. I have found that the adhesive doesn't stick as well. So, I will skip the shower for a day. If you don't feel comfortable with this, try showering the night before to allow the skin to dry before attaching the sensor.

Use two alcohol pads to clean the skin before application. In my experience, individually wrapped alcohol pads work better than using a paper towel and rubbing alcohol. Use the first pad to gently scrub the area of application. Scrub a larger area than the size of the sensor as you don't always get the sensor exactly where you want it. The second alcohol pad isn't for scrubbing so much as it is for removing what your scrub loosened. Natural oils, dirt, and loose skin cells can "noodle up" during the scrub part and prevent a firm attachment of the sensor if not removed. Once you have scrubbed and polished your area, let it air dry for at least a minute.

Position the device over the cleaned skin, then press quickly and firmly. The device will snap as it is pressure sensitive the moment you push it into your skin. Once it deploys, freeze. Just continue holding the device against your arm for a moment, then slowly rock the unit side to side before gently pulling the applicator off your arm. The sensor can sometimes stick to the applicator, and you don't want to accidentally lift an edge of the sensor when pulling the device away.

Gently press all around the edges of the sensor with your finger to further adhere the sticky pad to your skin.

Now that your sensor is installed, use your phone or reader to scan the sensor to activate it. Your sensor will need sixty minutes to set up before the first readings come in.

Note: On the first day of sensor use, I will be prompted to double check my blood sugars against my CGM sensor readings. I usually don't have to do this, but if my readings are low, I will.

When I used the FreeStyle Libre2 sensor and companion reader device, I found I needed to calibrate the two readings. The reader device is also a glucometer with its own test strips called FreeStyle Precision Neo. Occasionally on the first day, and sometimes on other days in the fourteen-day time period, my sensor's readings would be ridiculously off. I calibrated by using a test strip inserted into the FreeStyle reader device and a fingerstick. The results would display and then the next time I scanned the sensor on my arm, the previous "off" reading would begin to correct itself. With continual scans, the sensor number would approach the blood strip reading. Sometimes I'd have to do multiple blood strip readings over a few hours. This can feel like a pain in the batootie, but compared to not wearing a CGM and fingersticking multiple times a day instead, it is an acceptable displeasure for me.

That being said, The Freestyle Libre3 sensor doesn't need to be calibrated.

Some people have brought their sensor back to the pharmacy stating it wouldn't register on their reader, or it was broken in some other way. They got a dud. If this ever happens to you, call the phone number on the box or go to the company's website and request a new sensor. In my experience as a pharmacy technician, FreeStyle Libre has been really good about accommodating customers if the equipment is faulty.

I recommend you hold onto the empty box for the duration of the sensor. The outside of the box has the lot number printed on it and is usually asked for by FreeStyle Libre when reporting a defective sensor. I keep my empty box with my medications just in case I need to report a bad sensor. To date, I haven't ever needed to do that.

Removal of the sensor

The sensor's usage time has completed and now it's time to remove and attach a new one. If your sensor didn't lift away from your skin at all during the two weeks, you may find it tough to grasp an area to pull it away from your skin.

I've found if I use an alcohol pad and start loosening one spot of the adhesive pad on the sensor, I can lift a little bit and start the detachment process. I use the alcohol pad again, rubbing, dabbing, and allowing the alcohol to break down the adhesive. As I make my way around the perimeter of the sensor, separating the sensor pad from my skin, the filament pulls out of the skin. I haven't ever bled from removing a filament; however, there is sometimes dried blood on the underside of the sensor from insertion.

Your arm will most likely have a circle of gummy residue from the adhesive. Soap and water are not strong enough to remove the residue. Use a fresh alcohol pad to break down the bond. You can also use oils or lotions to help loosen the adhesive and rub it off, though it takes more time.

I haven't ever had a reaction to the FreeStyle Libre product line of adhesives, and I tend to react to low-quality adhesives. If you are worried about a skin reaction or have sensitive skin to other adhesive products, discuss that with your doctor before trying any product that uses adhesive.

Disposing of used sensors and application devices

The sensors have a battery inside, so you may want to group used sensors together and dispose of them with your other used batteries. The applicator devices are mostly hard plastic with a metal spring and needle inside. Check with your local waste management service to see if they accept the plastics involved for recycling. If so, take apart the applicator and remove the spring and needle. Put the needle in your sharps container and dispose of the spring.

CHAPTER 14: HOW TO READ THE RESULTS

If you treat your CGM as a training device when it comes to foods, you'll be able to learn what quantities of foods you can eat and still remain in your green zone.

The first time you wear a CGM, you'll need to know a few things about the numbers and graphs the device displays. The biggest, most important thing to know is it's natural to feel overwhelmed at first. You're going to see a lot of ups and downs on your graph, which is normal. Our bodies are in a constant balancing act concerning glucose levels, releasing insulin to help clear the glucose out of the bloodstream and into the cells, and then releasing glucagon when the sugar level drops to stimulate the liver to release some stored glucose to bring our numbers back up.

The glucose rollercoaster: Interstitial fluids verses blood glucose

Food is converted into glucose in the gut and absorbed into the blood which then travels all over the body and into the cells, some of which are in the interstitial layer just under the skin. (That's where your CGM filament is placed.) There is a time gap between food absorption and interstitial delivery. Think about a rollercoaster. You could sit in the front seat or the back seat. Both are on the same ride, but both seats do not crest the top of the hill at the same time. By the time the back seat reaches the top, the front seat is on its way down and the same goes for when the back seat is traveling through the bottom of the dip—the front seat is on its way up another hill. Our bodies are extremely efficient and can transport the glucose rather quickly, but there is a slight delay in the two readings after a meal. That's why there are arrows next to the numbers on CGM results.

The arrows let you know the direction the blood glucose is probably heading to give you an indication of how to treat your levels. Also, let's say your sensor reading says that you're below 70. Before you consume some sugar to bring your numbers up, pay attention to the arrow by the number. If it's a straight down arrow, that means you're still dropping in your blood glucose levels. A slightly angled arrow pointing down means your blood levels are slowing their descent. Horizontal arrows indicate leveling off. An angled arrow pointing upward means your blood sugar is beginning to climb, and a straight up arrow is a rapid climb.

Keep in mind, these arrows are not perfect. They should not be relied upon 100%. They are guides to help you understand what might be happening within your blood measurement. Remember, CGMs are not registering blood glucose, but interstitial fluid glucose.

If your reading is 69 with a straight down arrow, you might want to take your glucose tablets, (whatever amount your doctor recommends) and also test your blood with a fingerstick. But if you are 69 and the arrow is angled or horizontal, you could still check your blood to see where the number is, or you could wait a couple minutes to see where your sensor number goes. I have eaten carbs too many times, thinking I need to raise my blood sugar, but the front of the "rollercoaster" was already on its way back up and my consumed carbs pushed me up even further, more than I needed.

The fasting blood glucose level and your CGM reading should be fairly similar. On the rollercoaster ride, this would be the point when the ride is almost over, and the track is flat. The front and back cars are at the same level. I've notated the number on my CGM right before a fasting blood draw and then compared the two numbers once I received my results. They've almost always been within a couple of points.

With a CGM, you get continuous readings of what is happening inside your body. Just remember that CGMs are tools to help you manage your diabetes. They are not to be relied upon 100%. They are to help you have better insight.

If you see a number that doesn't feel right, especially if it's low, but you feel fine, don't panic. Feel free to fingerstick to double check. Same as if you see a reading of 90 but you are shaking and nauseous, do a fingerstick to make sure you're not lower than what the reader says.

Remember that even glucometers and test strips are not 100% accurate, either. If your body is telling you your blood sugar is low, listen to it and act accordingly. If your CGM and glucometer readings don't reflect what you're feeling, sit down and ask for help. You may need medical attention.

CHAPTER 15: ALARMS

Setting the alarms

Most CGMs have alarms. Not all, but most. Currently, I wear a FreeStyle Libre3 which pairs with my phone. My numbers are constantly uploaded from my sensor to my phone, and I don't need to scan my sensor. If I keep my phone nearby and powered on, the data is collected in the app. Other versions of the FreeStyle Libre have reader devices that can be used instead of a phone app. That's up to you. Whichever you choose to use as your reader, there are three alarms based on sugar levels: 180, 70, and 55. The 55 alarm cannot be disabled. The other two can be silenced or even raised or lowered. The 55 alarm is the emergency alarm—hypoglycemia. It only makes sense that this alarm can't be deactivated, since it is a much more immediate threat to your health.

If I'm at work, I might disable the highest alarm to avoid having it go off while helping a customer. I don't need to know when my glucose is too high as I don't take insulin. The low alarm of 70 is sometimes disabled if I'm going into a quiet setting like the library. I can always peek at my current reading and monitor any lower moments instead of just waiting for the alarm to go off. However, the 55 alarm is crucial. If my 55 alarm goes off, I need to address that promptly. When you first begin to wear a CGM, I recommend you keep the programmable alarms enabled, to help you adjust to learning about spikes or lows.

To set alarms, go into the menu section and select alarms. From there, choose which alarms to turn on. Select the glucose level you want the alarm to alert for, then go back to the home screen.

Turning off an alarm

How do you turn off the alarm once it activates? It's simple. Unlock your phone (if it's locked). Open the app to the home screen. The alarm will stop beeping.

If I had forgotten to return to the app's home page the last time I was in the app, then I would need to do that now in order to turn off the alarm.

Tip: Always return to the home screen before closing out of the app. Also, place the app icon on your phone's home screen so you don't have to search for it while the alarm is sounding. The first time the alarm goes off can be jarring, but with proper preparation, you can quickly turn it off.

CHAPTER 16: TROUBLESHOOTING

I'll mention the issues that I've encountered while using my CGM. Refer to the manufacturer's website for a full list of troubleshooting topics.

You'll need to keep the reader (or phone with the app) and sensor near each other for the readings to work. I can have my phone in the same room and it will continually connect with my sensor, transferring the data. If I leave my phone in another room, the data stream stops, and eventually, the app will sound a chirping alarm to let you know it can't detect the sensor. When this happens, I open the app to the home screen and the alarm turns off.

I usually have my phone nearby at all times, so this is not a common problem for me. If you have a job or classroom with rules about having phones on your person, you'll need to make your boss or teacher aware that your phone is essential to monitor your sugars.

Also, you'll need to keep an eye on your battery charge for whatever device you choose to read your sensor. A dead phone/reader won't alert you to a hypoglycemic episode.

Cannot connect to the sensor with phone

When using the app on your phone to read the sensor, you'll need to first adjust your settings. The first time you set up a sensor, you need to enable the NFC in your phone's settings. You should be able to find this by going to settings and looking under connections. NFC is the setting used for making credit card payments with your phone like Apple Pay or Samsung Wallet. Once your phone is paired with a new sensor, no other phone can connect accidentally. I know this because both my husband and I wore FreeStyle Libre3 sensors at the same time and we tested to see if my phone would work on his sensor. Nothing. With more and more people wearing these devices, and with some sensors transmitting continually to the paired phone, one might worry about your data going to the wrong phone or reader. That won't happen due to the unique one-time coding that creates the link between your sensor and your reader.

Keep in mind, you can't switch readers during the fourteen-day sensor period from a phone to a handheld reader. Whichever device you use as a reader for your sensor, you must use it to finish the two weeks.

Bluetooth needs connecting

What do you do if you get a message saying Bluetooth needs connecting? Go to Settings, Connections, and enable or turn on Bluetooth. If the setting is turned on already, but you are still getting the message saying it's not, reboot your phone. That will usually fix it.

Sensor Error message

Occasionally, you'll get a sensor error message. I get this message when my sugar is changing rapidly, either up or down. If I am spiking and get this message, I wait for ten minutes, then try again. If I'm crashing and get the sensor error, I do a fingerstick, check my blood sugar, then respond accordingly. Sometimes, the fingerstick shows my number isn't as low as the device states. That's good. But not knowing for sure can lead to over-consuming glucose tablets or drinking orange juice when not needed.

The nuclear method

Just like other apps, sometimes you need to uninstall and reinstall the program to fix certain problems. I recommend you first connect your device (phone or reader) to Libreview.com (if you are using their products) and save your data before uninstalling.

Apps get updated often and you may be prompted to install the latest version of the app. Again, back up your data, then uninstall the old and install the new version.

CHAPTER 17: THREE TEST SUBJECTS

I wanted to investigate how others may react to a CGM, so I asked my husband and two sisters if they'd be willing to wear a device for two weeks. This wasn't an official study of any kind, but merely an effort to have three people who have never worn a CGM to try one out and give feedback.

Larry had already observed my experiences using a CGM to manage my diabetes, so it wasn't as if he didn't know anything going into it. As soon as his unit was activated, he started experimenting with food, bagels for breakfast being the first thing he tried. He doesn't usually eat breakfast because doing so makes him tired, he's told me. On that day, his fasting sugar was in the healthy range and the glucose peak after eating the bagel hit 140, but then his sugar plummeted quickly. The low alarm sounded, and a few minutes later, the critical alarm sounded. The CGM said his sugar was 53.

This was his first day wearing the device and only the first couple of hours of wear. In my experience, sometimes those initial numbers can be wrong. So, I had him check his blood sugar with my glucometer. Alarmingly, his blood glucose was also 53. Larry was experiencing hypoglycemia!

I looked at him and asked, "How do you feel?" I tried to keep my voice in check, so I didn't scare him. I know how *my* body feels when I'm that low.

He answered, "I'm tired. I just want to lay down. This is why I don't eat breakfast. It makes me feel like this."

"You should discuss this event with your doctor at your next appointment," I said, hoping he would do that. "Perhaps you should try eating protein with your carbs next time."

Larry agreed. He recovered from his hypo moment over the next hour, which we closely monitored using the CGM.

That evening we both consumed the same quantity of food—a healthy meal with moderate levels of carbohydrates—and we watched our two CGMs display the differences between our bodies. Larry's glucose peak hit 140, whereas mine hit 180. Larry's glucose returned to normal quickly, which was good to see considering the hypo moment he had that morning. Mine was slower.

Unfortunately, Larry knocked off his sensor on the doorframe after only three days. He felt really bad, so he refilled the prescription for another CGM and purchased a box of large bandages to cover the sensor and started again.

The two-week time frame revealed a lot about his body and how it handles carbohydrates. Using Libreview, he was able to see the fourteen days at a glance to recognize patterns in his sugar numbers. Larry usually eats once a day, following the OMAD (one meal a day) diet plan. He discovered he can fast all day and his numbers will hold steady in the upper 80's to low 90's. Then he can eat a day's worth of calories in the evening hours, including protein and carbs and not spike higher than 140, and also not crash on the other end like with his bagel hypoglycemic moment.

His glucose increases looked like little mounds, slow, controlled . . . normal. Yet, the finding that carbs alone cause him to crash indicates he has some glucose control issues that could become more pronounced if he doesn't address this.

Prior to wearing the CGM, Larry didn't know that his tired episodes were probably low glucose. This finding has helped him to be more careful with his food choices.

Sister #2. She is the one who has had hypoglycemic episodes most of her life. She knows that when she feels irritable and/or low energy, she needs sugar. A few years ago, she learned her A1c was increasing, and she has been actively addressing it with diet and exercise whenever possible.

Wearing the CGM, she was able to see a couple of instances where her sugar spiked above 180, then plummeted due to consuming too many carbs. She was also able to determine the sustained energy benefits of eating protein with carbs, and also how taking a walk after a meal helped slow the Yo-Yo effect of her glucose levels.

Unfortunately, sister #2 knocked off her sensor by accident five days in, so we couldn't get any more information. (Another example of the need to secure the device until you become used to it.)

Even with only five days of information, my sister was able to see in real time what her body was doing with the food she was consuming.

Sister #1 is diabetic and takes metformin. She owns a glucometer and has tested her sugar levels from time to time. She sees her doctor regularly to keep tabs on her A1c and medication levels. The first night after application her arm was sore, due to attaching the sensor in the evening. The low alarm kept going off even though her blood glucometer showed normal numbers. Remember the critical 55 alarm can't be disabled, so she was awakened a couple times through the night with false alarms. She told me that she felt like the sensor was loose, so she used a bandage to secure it. After that, the readings stopped being false alarms and showed more consistency with her blood levels. All we could figure was the filament wasn't deep enough to get a good reading, and by attaching the bandage, it pushed the filament further into the interstitial fluid.

Coincidentally, because of securing the sensor on the first night, she was able to keep it on for the full fourteen days.

Her findings over the two-week period were shocking as she became aware of which of the foods she regularly consumed made her sugar levels climb. Since then, she has tried to adopt healthier eating habits. In the end, she joked that she didn't like wearing the CGM because it revealed things she can't unsee. "I won't be able to enjoy graham crackers and milk anymore without remembering what they did to my sugar level. I thought the protein in the milk would help balance the carbs in the crackers. I was wrong."

Here is an example of how continuing to wear a CGM could help her experiment and establish what amounts of foods and snacks she should eat to keep her sugars manageable and individualized for her body. She could try the graham crackers and milk treat again but with fewer crackers, or maybe with some physical activity afterward, or possibly with some added protein. All of those experiments take time and patience but could be rewarding for her to discover how to best enjoy a treat while being diabetic.

CHAPTER 18: READY FOR THE NEXT STEP WITH A CGM?

Diabetes is a process. Many people struggle with it, as I have, and feel alone in their ups and downs. It can be overwhelming to think about drastic life changes, complications, and a lifetime commitment.

This is why I decided to write this book, to help minimize these fears and offer alternate support and solutions to a difficult and fluctuating illness.

With the help of CGM devices, and my diabetes toolbox, I was able to find a balance once again for my body. My CGM allows me to live with diabetes, not be hampered by it, by understanding what the foods I eat are doing to my glucose levels. You might think, yeah, but Lorena, your A1c kept climbing after starting to wear a CGM. Yes, it did, because of other factors at play at that time, including side effects and adjustments to medication. However, the data and information I gathered right from the start about the foods I like to eat still hold true today.

I encourage you to try adding a continuous glucose monitor to your diabetes toolbox, even if for just two weeks. Ask your doctor for a prescription and/or free sample, check online at FreeStyle Libre for a free trial coupon, or if you're financially able, pay out of pocket. (Don't forget to use GoodRx or any other online prescription discount company for a reduction in price.)

And secure the sensor with a large bandage right away.

You can change your future by managing your blood sugar today.

As a final note, I never realized my first novel, ***A Diamond in My Pocket*** has a plot point similar to this journey. The protagonist is given the ability, contained within a mystical diamond, to see the impending doomed future for her and her group. She sets out to make small changes in the present to alter the course of the futures of everyone in her life, basically to save lives.

With diabetes, the same holds true for what we can do for our own futures. We can make small changes, a little at a time, and see the positive results from what may have seemed like a bleak outlook.

For myself, I use my CGM and toolbox to guide me on my diabetic journey, giving me the power to set my future. It's a future I'm looking forward to.

I'm optimistic you'll consider doing the same.

EPILOGUE

Writing a book takes time, and during the time completing this book, I had a medical incident (gastrointestinal) that put me in the emergency room. Following that event, I stopped taking Ozempic as per medical advice from my PA. The intent was to wait a few months for my body to return to normal and then restart it because of the amazing blood sugar control I had experienced. However, as the months ticked by, and by using my CGM, I could see my body wasn't returning to normal. Therefore, I haven't started Ozempic again as of March 2024. And yes, my A1c has climbed. But as I stated earlier in the book, I can see exactly what is happening in real time and with each food choice that I put into my body.

My diabetes journey continues, and perhaps I'll write another book about my medical event that altered the way I treat my diabetes and has set me on a course of new discoveries. One thing remains the same, though, my CGM lights the way through the fog, keeping me in check, and reminding me of unhealthy choices so I can evaluate, restructure, and continue being resilient.

Additionally, Dexcom announced that coming in the summer of 2024, they will release an over-the-counter CGM available for non-insulin patients to purchase without a prescription. Abbott has already released an OTC version in the UK, available without a prescription.

The world is jumping on the CGM bandwagon, and I'm absolutely excited!

THANK YOU

Thank you so much for purchasing my book. I hope you've felt encouraged, supported, and are now armed with new knowledge of how you want to progress forward along your diabetic journey.

Before you go, if you enjoyed the book, **would you please consider posting a review on the platform where you purchased it?** Posting a review is the best and easiest way to support the work of independent authors like me.

Your feedback will help me to keep writing the kind of books that will help you get the results you want. It would mean a lot to me to hear from you.

Also, please feel free to visit my website at www.CGMtips.com and join my email list. You'll be notified when new books are released, along with new videos and blog posts about diabetes.

Visit LorenaAngell.com to see my fiction books.

REFERENCES

Any information that was not from my personal experiences were found from the following reference materials:

Centers for Disease Control and Prevention – www.CDC.gov/diabetes

National Institutes of Health – www.NIH.gov

American Diabetes Association – www.diabetes.org

References:

[1] Melanoma and diabetes

Dobrică, E., Banciu, M. L., Kipkorir, V., Tabari, M. a. K., Cox, M. J., Kutikuppala, L. S., & Găman, M. (2022). Diabetes and skin cancers: Risk factors, molecular mechanisms and impact on prognosis. *World Journal of Clinical Cases, 10*(31), 11214–11225.

https://doi.org/10.12998/wjcc.v10.i31.11214

URL=https://pubmed.ncbi.nlm.nih.gov/36387789/

[2]

Laursen, J. C., Jepsen, R., Bruun-RasmuSsen, N. E., Frimodt-Møller, M., Jørgensen, M. E., Persson, F., & Hansen, C. S. (2022). Blood oxygen saturation is lower in persons with pre-diabetes and screen-detected diabetes compared with non-diabetic individuals: A population-based study of the Lolland-Falster Health Study cohort. *Frontiers in Epidemiology*, *2*. https://doi.org/10.3389/fepid.2022.1022342

[3] Interfering Substances & Procedures for CGMs

Diabetes Care & Education. (n.d.). ADCES. https://diabeteseducator.org/

[4]

Ahmed, M. H., Barakat, S., & Almobarak, A. O. (2014). The association between renal stone disease and cholesterol gallstones: the easy to believe and not hard to retrieve theory of the metabolic syndrome. *Renal Failure*, *36*(6), 957–962. https://doi.org/10.3109/0886022x.2014.900424
Full article: The association between renal stone disease and cholesterol gallstones: the easy to believe and not hard to retrieve theory of the metabolic syndrome (tandfonline.com)

AUTHOR BIO

Lorena Angell writes fiction and non-fiction, having first published in 2011 after hearing the encouraging quote, "You won't know unless you try."

For fiction, she writes YA urban fantasy inspired one night while dreaming. Ms. Angell's first book A DIAMOND IN MY POCKET, book one of eight in The Unaltered Series, quickly soared up the Movers & Shakers chart. iTunes iBookstore recognized POCKET as a Breakout Book, and subsequent titles in The Unaltered Series have all reached #1 in their categories on Amazon, which helped her procure option rights for the series for film and television.

Ms. Angell also writes romantic suspense with her series Lost Crown. ROYAL REFUGEE, the first in the trilogy, follows a family's defiance of a neighboring country's dictator by hiding and assisting the refugees fleeing the oppressive regime. It was a semifinalist in Kindle Book Review's 2020 Young Adult category.

As for non-fiction, after being diagnosed with insulin resistance in 2007, Ms. Angell endured a health journey that she believes many people can relate to. She wrote her memoir-esque story with the hopes of helping others who may have struggled as well, using her experience as a pharmacy technician and her trial-and-error with medications and devices as an added background for the book. She also created and published daily diabetes journals to help others track their blood sugar levels.

In her downtime, Ms. Angell enjoys barbequing, gardening, reading, and learning how to make the perfect cup of espresso. She lives in southwest Washington with her husband and their cat named Squirrel.

Made in United States
Troutdale, OR
09/24/2026

54818414R00090